Selenium

Selenium

Are You Getting Enough to Reduce Your Risk of Cancer?

Edgar N. Drake, Ph.D.

Writer's Showcase
San Jose New York Lincoln Shanghai

Selenium
Are You Getting Enough to Reduce Your Risk of Cancer?

Writer's Showcase
an imprint of iUniverse.com, Inc.

For information address:
iUniverse.com, Inc.
5220 S 16th, Ste. 200
Lincoln, NE 68512
www.iuniverse.com

This book is written solely for information. It is not intended as medical advice or as an alternative to the counsel of your physician. No change in your dietary regimen should be undertaken without the prior approval of your physician.

This book presents evidence that dietary selenium supplements can prevent a substantial fraction of cancers from occurring in populations of people, but does not state, imply, or guarantee that cancers can be prevented in any given person. Nothing in the title or contents of this book is intended to suggest that dietary selenium supplementation will prevent, treat, or cure cancer in any specific person.

ISBN: 0-595-18066-3

Printed in the United States of America

Dedication

*This book is dedicated with love
to my wife, Nina,
who nurtures and enriches my life
and to my children Ginger, Dana, and Ed
who inspire me with their accomplishments.*

Table of Contents

Preface

Someone had to write this book. How else could you know that something as simple, easy, and inexpensive as dietary supplementation with the essential mineral selenium could significantly improve the chances of you or your loved ones avoiding the terrible suffering and expense of cancer? Neatly hidden away in scientific journals are no fewer than three decades of sound epidemiological studies, animal cancer-prevention experiments, *in vitro* human cancer cell studies, and successful clinical trials in the United States and China, which collectively attest to the cancer-preventive effectiveness of selenium.

Although there have been many books extolling the health benefits of specific dietary supplements, a disappointingly large number have proven to be without scientific basis and, appropriately, have been either criticized or dismissed by the medical establishment. Biomedical research scientists and physicians involved in academic medicine are quite accomplished at discriminating between nutrients that have real health benefits and "snake oil." Unfortunately, 99.9% of the human population is not included in these groups and is significantly less able to make such distinctions.

The pace of biomedical discoveries has become so great that it is difficult even for the researchers themselves to stay current in their areas of expertise. With the exploding volume of valid, peer-reviewed scientific and medical research publications, it is unrealistic to expect practicing physicians to be familiar with the most recent discoveries in all areas affecting human health such as trace element nutrition.

The layperson, lacking both the time and the training to access and read the technical literature with understanding, is constrained to depend on the mass media for nutritional information. The variety and "sound byte" nature of news reports is such that we may have heard about selenium, but we have little real understanding of what it is and its importance to us. Unlike drugs, the sale of most individual nutritional supplements is not sufficiently profitable for manufacturers to promote their products through the various advertising media.

Literally hundreds of companies produce diets, vitamins, minerals, and herbs to take advantage of our pervasive nutritional ignorance. In an effort to determine which products actually contribute to improving the quality of our lives, we normally depend upon those we trust—our families or close friends. However well meaning, these individuals typically are not nutritional researchers and are not sufficiently informed to offer sound opinions regarding specific dietary components. Vague or conflicting answers from those we consult do not instill confidence and, too often, we opt for choices that are unsupported by data.

In adopting the responsibility for writing this book, I understand my task to be two-fold. First, I must write a clear (i.e. as free as possible of esoteric scientific jargon) and compelling yet concise presentation of the facts sufficient for any layperson to make an informed personal decision concerning dietary selenium supplementation. Secondly, the information presented must be credible to the scientific and medical communities. The latter requirement means that crucial statements must be documented by citations in the peer-reviewed scientific and medical literature. Rather than relying solely upon my deliberately succinct presentation of the relevant facts, physicians, scientists, other health professionals, and individuals interested in perusing the original research papers can access the primary literature citations. Omission of such references is a tacit admission that the writing has no basis in fact.

It is critically important for the reader to understand that the various chemical forms of naturally-occurring selenium differ greatly in the way they are metabolized in humans and, therefore, in their cancer-preventive effectiveness. The sound scientific evidence for the cancer-preventive efficacy of the several dietary forms of selenium is presented in Chapter 3, but necessarily requires some chemical vocabulary more familiar to physicians and scientists. Chapters 4 and 5 detail the biochemical evidence that constitutes the basis for an understanding of how selenium exerts its cancer-preventive effects. The information in Chapters 3, 4 and 5, while admittedly somewhat technical, is essential to achieving a sufficient degree of credibility from scientists and physicians. Lay readers who prefer to know only the practical significance of the evidence presented may skip these chapters or postpone their reading until more time can be allocated to in-depth study.

Acknowledgements

By the time their books finally appear in print, most authors have received many valuable contributions from a considerable number of people. It is always with much gratitude that we recognize those who have helped us improve the quality of our work.

In my case, I must start by thanking my wife for her continuous support, encouragement, opinions, grammatical expertise and, especially, her patience. Spouses often pay a high price for their mate's literary adventures.

The critical reading of a manuscript requires a substantial commitment of time and thought. To be of value to the author, the reader also must be willing to express his honest appraisal of the work. This book has been improved greatly by the thoughtful comments and suggestions of Mary Berg, David Crockett, Jack Dinsmoor, Fazlur Rahman, M.D., Beryle Williams, and William Williams. I am very grateful for their insights.

Introduction

This book is written solely for information. It is not intended as medical advice or as an alternative to the counsel of your physician. No change in your dietary regimen should be undertaken without the prior approval of your physician.

This book presents evidence that dietary selenium supplements can prevent a substantial fraction of cancers from occurring in populations of people, but does not state, imply, or guarantee that cancers can be prevented in any given person. Nothing in the title or contents of this book is intended to suggest that dietary selenium supplementation will prevent, treat, or cure cancer in any specific person.

CHAPTER 1

CANCER FACTS: THE PROMISE OF PREVENTION

"What are the facts? Again and again and again—what are the facts? Shun wishful thinking, ignore divine revelation, forget what 'the stars foretell,' avoid opinion, care not what the neighbors think, never mind the unguessable 'verdict of history'—what are the facts and to how many decimal places? You pilot always into an unknown future; facts are your single clue. Get the facts!"

Robert A. Heinlein

Introduction

Studies published in the scientific and medical literature report that selenium, the naturally-occurring mineral produced by volcanic eruptions, prevents human cancer when taken daily in appropriately large amounts. According to the Center for Disease Control (CDC), cancer is the second leading killer disease in the United States. Faced with the preceding statements, it appears illogical that most Americans are not employing the simple, safe, and inexpensive expedient of taking dietary selenium supplements to insure that their intakes are sufficient to prevent cancer. The savings, in terms of both human suffering and expense, would be prodigious. The explanation appears to be a slow, inefficient, and piecemeal dissemination of new scientific discoveries that is related to a financial disincentive to our health care system. To be sure, there are other reasons.

The present chapter explains that most cancers result from our repeated exposures to larger-than-average amounts of both natural and man-made cancer-causing substances (carcinogens) rather than individual genetic differences that produce familial predispositions. Implicit in understanding that most cancers have environmental causes is the realization that we can prevent the greatest majority from occurring.

When we appreciate that many carcinogens originate from natural rather than man-made sources, then we are able to understand that they occur everywhere and cannot be avoided. Indeed, our success in preventing cancer is dependent upon the knowledge that it is the amount of carcinogen we encounter rather than its presence per se that is critically important. Thus, of necessity, our goal is to minimize, rather than eliminate, our exposure to carcinogens.

In an exactly analogous way, we can choose diets and dietary supplements that maximize our intake of anticarcinogens (those substances that prevent and/or in some way inhibit cancer)—but only if we know what they are. That the anticarcinogen selenium occurs naturally, albeit in small amounts in our food, accounts for the fact that its cancer-preventing properties are not general knowledge. Products consisting of naturally-occurring substances cannot be protected by patents. Pharmaceutical companies cannot invest large sums of money in unprotected products. Moreover, the financial interest of the clear majority of professional health care providers resides in treatment rather than the prevention of disease. Absent any financial incentive, it is unrealistic to expect the health care industry to know much about or promote dietary supplementation with selenium. It should come as no surprise that treatment of disease with drugs gets more press than prevention of disease with dietary supplements or more reasoned food selections.

On Christmas day in 1996, the *Journal of the American Medical Association* published the results of a decade-long, clinical trial in which modest dietary selenium supplements reduced total cancer incidence among seniors in the U.S. by 37%. In terms of human lives impacted, this figure amounts to approximately 480,000 Americans who could be saved from the suffering and expense of cancer annually. The statistically significant reduction was accomplished without other changes in diet, exercise, or lifestyle. A single, daily, 200-microgram, selenium supplement alone was sufficient. Furthermore, the impressive result was achieved with no reports of toxicity.

The peer-review scientific and medical literature is published solely on the basis of merit, with no financial bias or agenda, and, thus, constitutes our best source of objective and reliable information. Those of us in the baby boomer-and-up age group have no time to wait for everyone to become informed and to reach a consensus concerning dietary selenium supplementation. Rather, we are best served by acquainting ourselves with the state-of-the-art scientific data and calling them to the attention of our primary care physicians.

Cancer in the United States

The threat of cancer occupies a place in all our minds when we reach middle age in the United States. We know that some 600,000 Americans die each year from cancer in the face of the world's most advanced and sophisticated health care system. We know that back in 1971, President Nixon "declared war on cancer" when he signed into law the National Cancer Act. We know that the National Cancer Institute (NCI) has spent approximately $34 billion between 1971 and 1996 fighting this disease. We also know that after our substantial investments of intellectual and financial resources, we are experiencing increased incidences of lung cancer in women, liver cancer, melanoma, multiple myeloma, non-Hodgkin's lymphoma, as well as esophageal, prostate, and kidney cancers. According to the National Cancer Institute, cancer is the second leading cause of death in the United States, and people in the 55-and-up age group account for 90% of the 1.3 million new cancer cases occurring annually. Indeed, our national cancer statistics make the disease appear so formidable that we are resigned to live with it much as we do with the threats of global nuclear war, the Ebola virus, or large asteroids impacting the earth.

You Must Determine Your Personal Cancer Risk

Our investment in research has bought us considerable insight into the process of carcinogenesis (the beginning of cancer). Armed with this knowledge, we can reduce our cancer risk to the degree that **it is not a practical concern**. It is known, for example, that to develop cancer, the cells of our bodies must be exposed to carcinogens (cancer-causing substances) or carcinogenic radiations (ultraviolet light, x-rays, and radiations from radioactive isotopes). It is also a fact that our cells are protected from becoming cancerous by assimilating anticarcinogens (substances which prevent or interfere with carcinogenesis). With a little knowledge, we can minimize our exposure to carcinogens and maximize our contacts with anticarcinogens. In so doing, we can reduce significantly our risks of this terrible disease. Our success in preventing cancer depends upon our choices of places to live and work as well as what we eat, drink, and breathe. Learning how to protect our cells from becoming cancerous is easy, and the reward for doing so is immeasurably great.

Over twenty years ago, Sir Richard Doll, Professor of Medicine at Oxford University and internationally recognized cancer researcher (Doll 1977), wrote: "…the evidence that cancer can be prevented has accumulated steadily and is now overwhelming…we should be able to reduce age-specific incidence rates—which account for one-quarter of all deaths of men in Britain under 75 years of age—by at least 80 to 90%." Tobacco and dietary choices account for the majority of cancer cases in the United States. The use of tobacco in all its forms is responsible for an estimated 30% of our cancer cases (Greenwald and Sondik 1986a), and dietary preferences cause another 35% (Doll and Peto 1981). Other risk factors, including occupational exposure to carcinogens and genetic predisposition to certain cancers, account for some 10% of total cancer incidence (Greenwald and Sondik 1986b) and (Knudson 1977).

If all of us decided to stop using tobacco in any form, the number of cancer cases in the United States each year would be reduced by about 390,000! If we add to that the cancer cases avoided from people choosing low-risk diets, the total number of cancer cases prevented annually increases to 845,000! The amount of money and human suffering saved by eliminating these two risk factors alone is incalculably large.

Certainly, it has not been made clear what constitutes a low-risk cancer diet. Obviously, the consumption of certain foods must be reduced while other foods, as well as certain vitamins and minerals, should be eaten in greater amounts. With all the recent claims about the strides made in understanding cancer, there has been an annoyingly small number of recommendations with respect to specific foods, vitamins, and minerals in amounts that are appropriate for a low-risk diet for cancer.

Calories, Fat, and Alcohol

There is some general agreement about specific dietary choices that contribute to increasing our cancer risk. In their 1996 report, "Carcinogens and Anticarcinogens in the Human Diet" (National Research Council 1996), the Committee on Comparative Toxicity of Naturally Occurring Carcinogens of the National Research Council identifies three dietary factors that correlate strongly with cancer incidence: total calories, fat content, and amount of alcohol consumed. The main culprit is fat. Since fat contains 225% of the calories by weight of either carbohydrates or proteins, a high-fat diet is synonymous with a high-calorie diet. Fats, particularly unsaturated fats, tend to combine with oxygen in our cells to produce high-energy, chemically-active substances that can damage our cellular DNA and may initiate the transformation from normal to malignant cells.

Dietary Fat and the U.S. Obesity Epidemic

That high-fat diets and high-cancer risk occur together is not good news for the typical American. We **love** the taste of fat! In many families with both husband and wife working outside the home, it is tempting and very convenient to eat meals out on workdays. In the competitive restaurant industry, businesses often maintain their market share by serving delicious, high-fat food. Even salads and vegetables served in cafeterias frequently are prepared with high-fat garnishes to enhance their flavor. Our ignorance of the fat content of restaurant food allows us to enjoy a savory meal without being concerned about obesity or any associated cancer risk (a low-guilt diet).

As reported in a fairly recent issue of the journal *Science* (Taubes 1998), data from the National Health and Nutrition Examination Survey (NHANES) show that 54% of the United States adult population are overweight and 23% are obese. Furthermore, 25% of children are either overweight or obese. A comparison of the current data with previous surveys is sobering. NHANES data show that obesity in U.S. adults has increased from 12.8% in 1962 to 14.8% in 1980 to 22.5% in 1994. An estimated 60 million persons are affected with some degree of obesity, which causes some 300,000 deaths per year and an economic loss of $50 to $100 billion per year.

Alcohol

The stereotypical American is an aggressive, work-weary person trying to manage a fast-paced, high-pressure lifestyle. Business is often conducted at lunch over drinks while "happy hour" and cocktail parties afford relaxation and stress reduction at the end of the day. Traditionally, alcohol has been the lubricant used to reduce friction between fast-living people.

In their 749-page report, "Diet and Health: Implications for Reducing Chronic Disease Risk" (National Research Council 1989), the Committee on Diet and Health, Food and Nutrition Board of the National Research Council concluded that excessive alcohol consumption, especially by individuals using tobacco or those with poor diets, was associated with an increased incidence of several types of cancer. In addition, the International Agency for Research on Cancer (IARC) has classified any alcoholic beverage as a "known carcinogen."

With fat and alcohol serving as staples in the American diet for decades, it is not terribly surprising that cancer ranks second only to heart disease as the most important killer disease in the United States. Happily, the increased public awareness of the connections between high-fat diets, heart disease, and cancer has prompted food manufacturers to produce an increasingly greater number of low-fat and fat-free alternatives to their original products. Although public concern over the composition of our foods should be viewed as a positive thing, we need to be better informed so that we can address only valid concerns and not waste our time, energy, and money on invalid worries.

Unwarranted Cancer Concerns

People in the business of selling health foods or food supplements have learned about the marketing power of the words "natural" and "organic," and the negative connotations associated with the word "chemical." These words are misunderstood so generally when applied to nutrition that I want to devote a bit of text to clarify their meaning and significance.

"Natural" is that occurring in nature. In terms of food components, it implies vitamins, minerals, carbohydrates, proteins, fats, herbs, etc. as they are found in a particular environment or matrix such as fruits, vegetables, or meat. The alternatives to natural food components are referred to as "synthetic" because they have been synthesized (manufactured) by a chemist in some laboratory. The public understands man-made substances to be "chemicals." Scientists and physicians all understand that all substances, whether natural or man-made, are chemicals. Food supplements are really not foods, but food components. Natural supplements are advertised as being superior to synthetic ones just because they are components of our natural foods. The philosophy is that our bodies have evolved in contact with naturally-occurring foods and, thereby, are adapted to the exposure. In fact, physicians often argue that food supplements should not be taken in lieu of the very same components found in food; their argument is that there might be some other component in the food that enhances the benefit of the nutrient.

Chemists understand the word "natural" as it is used in describing food supplements such as vitamins, etc. to mean the chemical form (i.e. the compound or isomer) that occurs naturally. For our purposes here, we may consider compounds as different combinations of elements. For example, magnesium sulfate (epsom salt) and magnesium hydroxide (milk of magnesia) are different compounds and are, therefore, different chemical forms of the element magnesium. Isomers are substances that have identical numbers and kinds of elements combined together, but the elements are connected together differently. For example, vitamin C (ascorbic acid) consists of six carbon atoms, eight hydrogen atoms, and six oxygen atoms all connected together. Thus, vitamin C is always represented by the formula $C_6H_8O_6$. However, there are two kinds of ascorbic acid, d-ascorbic acid and l-ascorbic acid, differing only in the directions certain atoms point in space. Organisms do not make d-ascorbic acid so that citrus fruits, broccoli, cauliflower, and other foods containing ascorbic acid always contain only l-ascorbic acid. Natural ascorbic acid, therefore, is l- rather than d-ascorbic acid.

Chemists also understand that all l-ascorbic acid, whether manufactured by a plant or a chemist in some laboratory, is identical in every particular. So it is technically correct to call l-ascorbic acid manufactured in a laboratory "natural." You should understand that a bottle labeled "natural vitamin C with rose hips" could legitimately be synthetic l-ascorbic acid to which a little bit of rose hips has been added.

The *American Collegiate Dictionary* defines the meaning of the word "organic" as follows: "noting or pertaining to a class of chemical compounds which formerly comprised only those existing in or derived from living organisms (animal or plant), but which now includes these and all other compounds of carbon." All scientists subscribe to this definition. By contrast, the general public understands "organic" to mean "grown without pesticides, antibiotics, or synthetic fertilizers." Our concerns about synthetic (man-made) pesticides such as Chlordane and Heptachlor and the cancer risks they pose can be measured by the amount of "organic" produce sold. Sales of "organic" vegetables have risen from some $2 billion in 1980 to approximately $6 billion in 1996. The growing popularity of synthetic-pesticide-free gardening is evidence of one of the widespread misconceptions concerning the cancer risks posed by synthetic pesticides in our food supply. Somehow, it escapes us that plants cannot run away from the insects that feed upon them and, therefore, must have adapted themselves for protection from insects in order to survive. In their evolution, plants developed the ability to make their own pesticides, fungicides, and repellents. Many of these natural food components are carcinogens! Caffeic acid, which is a natural component of many fruits and vegetables (especially abundant in apples and lettuce), is identified as a carcinogen by the International Agency for Research on Cancer (IARC). Estragole, a compound found in oil of tarragon as well as the herbs basil and fennel, is a carcinogen. Other examples include: tannic acid in teas, wine, coffee, and cocoa; allyl isothiocyanate in mustard, horseradish, and garlic; safrole in nutmeg and mace; psoralens in parsley and celery; hydrazines in mushrooms; and symphytine in comfrey tea. Whether or not those who buy "organic" vegetables are aware of it, their very expensive produce contains **natural carcinogens!**

The matter of cancer risk posed by pesticides in our foods has been evaluated extensively by scientists. Dr. Bruce N. Ames in the Division of Biochemistry and Molecular Biology at the University of California at Berkeley estimates that among plant pesticides, 99.99% are natural rather than synthetic (Ames, Profet, and Gold 1990). On the basis of weight, the amounts of natural pesticides in plants are 10,000 times as great as those synthesized by man (Snyder 1995). In February, 1996, the National Research Council of the National Academy of Sciences issued a report entitled "Carcinogens and Anticarcinogens in the Human Diet: A Comparison of Naturally-Occurring and Synthetic Substances" (National Research Council 1996). The report states that approximately 25% of all cancers are caused by our diet and that the natural carcinogens in foods greatly outnumber synthetic carcinogens. Most importantly, the Council further concluded that both natural and synthetic carcinogens are consumed at sufficiently low levels that **neither is likely to pose a cancer threat to humans.**

Why Don't The Carcinogens in Our Food Cause Cancer?

In our information-intensive society, almost daily we hear that more and more substances cause cancer. Bombarded as we are with such scary news, many of us have adopted the attitude, "Everything causes cancer so why worry about it?" This fatalistic response is understandable for the greatest number of people who do not understand that cancer risk is determined by the **amount of carcinogen** present—**not its presence per se.** All physicians and scientists know that chemical harm and benefit depend critically upon the dose. Whether substances are natural or synthetic, there are safe and unsafe amounts of exposure (Ottoboni 1991).

Much scientific effort is devoted to determining safe amounts of all substances. The United States Food and Drug Administration requires all pharmaceutical companies to establish the safety of their products. The dose of all chemicals, including carcinogens, depends upon their biological potency. An outstanding example is posed by the naturally-occurring carcinogen aflatoxin B_1. While liver cancer is relatively uncommon in the United States, it is one of the most prevalent kinds of cancer in Kenya, Swaziland, and Mozambique. The high incidence of liver cancer in these countries is attributable to aflatoxin B_1, which is produced by the fungus *Aspergillis Flavus*, and grows on corn, wheat, and peanuts, especially in hot, damp climates. Aflatoxin B_1 is the most potent carcinogen ever tested in animal experiments. A little detective work revealed that the incidence of liver cancer in these countries occurred in proportion to the amount of aflatoxin B_1 measured in their food supplies. Of course, corn, peanuts, and wheat in the United States also contain aflatoxin B_1. Fortunately, our food-handling techniques keep aflatoxin B_1 levels below those that would constitute a significant cancer risk to humans. The fact that liver cancer is a minor disease in the United States is encouraging evidence that we can achieve safe levels of even the most potent carcinogens.

That many of the carcinogens we encounter in our foods and environments are well known enables us to reduce our exposure to these substances. We know, for example, that benzo(a)pyrene is a potent carcinogen in cigarette smoke and smoke from our backyard barbecue grills. Grilling chicken, fish, or beef converts some of the nitrogen-containing substances in the meat into 2-amino-1-methyl-6-phenylimidazo[4,5-b]pyridine (PhIP), a carcinogen that has been shown to produce cancers in both large and small intestines of male rats and breast cancers in female rats. Dimethylnitrosoamine is one of the carcinogens formed from the amines in our bodies combining with sodium nitrite, a bactericide added to bacon, hot dogs, and lunchmeat to prevent poisoning from botulism toxin. Foods prepared from fermentation such as bread, yogurt, and alcoholic beverages contain the naturally-occurring carcinogen urethane, which has been proven to cause a variety of cancers in mice, rats, and hamsters. Chloroform is one of several carcinogens produced when we chlorinate our public water supplies. If we live in an area where the surface geology is granite, then the air in our homes contains radon, a carcinogen that can produce lung cancer. In the mountains where there is less atmosphere to protect us from the sun's high-energy radiation, we must use sunscreen to protect ourselves from the increased risk of the skin cancers basal cell carcinoma, squamous cell carcinoma, and melanoma. If we choose to smoke, barbeque often, expose our skin to the sun, eat large quantities of prepared meats, adopt a high-fat diet, or drink alcohol excessively, we are increasing the amounts of carcinogens we encounter, and thereby, are opting for a greater cancer risk.

Learning about Anticarcinogens

We can substantially reduce our risk of most cancers by consuming larger amounts of anticarcinogens. Anticarcinogens are substances that interfere with the initiation, promotion, or progression of cancer. These substances are found primarily in fruits and vegetables, and like carcinogens, may be either natural or synthetic. Flavones, indoles, phenols, isocyanates, and coumarins are several types of anticarcinogens that occur naturally in plants. Examples of synthetic anticarcinogens are BHA (butylated hydroxyanisole) and BHT (butylated hydroxytoluene). Cruciferous vegetables such as broccoli, Brussels sprouts, cabbage, and cauliflower contain certain indoles including indole-3-carbinol, 3,3'-diindolymethane, and indole-3-acetonitrile. Both flavones and indoles inhibit benzo(a)pyrene-induced cancers in mice. Indole-3-carbinol and 3,3'-diiodolymethane also inhibit the formation of dimethylbenzanthracene-induced breast cancers in rats.

The optimal low-cancer-risk diet then is one that maximizes the amounts of anticarcinogens while minimizing the amounts of carcinogens. It is precisely for this reason that The American Cancer Society (ACS) recommends that we eat generous amounts of fruits and vegetables while limiting our intakes of fat and alcohol.

The Scientific Determination of Cancer Risk

The mere presence of carcinogens or anticarcinogens in our food, whether natural or synthetic, does not establish that they are having any measurable effect on our cancer risk. The amounts of carcinogens and anticarcinogens needed for foods to have minimal cancer risk must be determined experimentally. The three methods used to determine the doses of carcinogens and anticarcinogens necessary to have an effect upon cancer risk are epidemiological studies, animal studies, and clinical trials.

Epidemiological studies are designed to answer the question, "Do certain things occur together?" The fact that certain cancers are more prevalent in some geographic areas than others suggests that some environmental factor may be causing the effect. In the case of liver cancer mentioned earlier, one might ask, "Do people with larger amounts of aflatoxin B_1 in their foods have a greater incidence of liver cancer?" If an epidemiological study shows that the answer is yes, the **possibility** of a cause-and-effect relationship between aflatoxin B_1 and liver cancer is established. The fact that larger amounts of dietary aflatoxin B_1 and liver cancer occur together does not **prove** that aflatoxin B_1 causes liver cancer. The proof that any specific amount of dietary aflatoxin B_1 results in human cancer could only be demonstrated by feeding human subjects food containing aflatoxin B_1, which obviously could not be done. The best alternative is an animal study in which one group of animals is given food with a specific dose of aflatoxin B_1, and a second group is fed an identical diet except that it is free of aflatoxin B_1. If a cause-and-effect relationship is found in laboratory animals, the minimum dose necessary to produce the effect can be established.

In those experiments designed to identify anticarcinogens, double blind, placebo-controlled clinical trials are most conclusive. In a typical study, cancer-free human research subjects are randomly divided into two groups: those receiving a specific dose of a dietary supplement and those receiving a placebo (a substance with no known effect upon cancer). When a sufficiently large number of subjects is studied for a sufficiently long time, any differences in the cancer incidences can be detected and the anticarcinogenic effectiveness of the particular supplement can be evaluated. Double blind means that neither the research subjects nor the researcher measuring the results knows which subjects are receiving the dietary supplement so that bias is eliminated. Since human clinical trials often involve hundreds of research subjects studied for a decade of time, they tend to be extraordinarily expensive and, therefore, few in number.

Before the results of any study are widely accepted by the scientific and medical communities as established fact, they must be independently replicated. Sometimes scientific studies produce apparently conflicting results that are attributable to various factors including experimental design. When seemingly contradictory results are made public by the media, people who do not understand that scientific fact emerges from the collective knowledge of many studies become confused and cynical.

Exciting Cancer News

The purpose of this book is to make as many people as possible aware of the huge body of scientific and medical literature that supports the contention that dietary supplementation with the anticarcinogenic mineral selenium can lower the risk of human cancer. The anticarcinogenic properties of both natural and synthetic selenium compounds have been thoroughly and systematically investigated for the past 30 years. Every four years since 1976, scientists have held an international symposium on the role of selenium in biology and medicine. There have been many epidemiological studies in the United States, Finland, and China, all of which have indicated that greater dietary intakes of selenium are associated with lower incidences of cancer in these countries. There have been scores of animal studies, which have repeatedly demonstrated that laboratory animals can be protected from cancers induced by either viruses or carcinogens by simply supplementing their diets with non-toxic doses of several naturally occurring anticarcinogenic selenium compounds. As if giving the world a Christmas present, Dr. Larry Clark, et al., published the results of their ten-year, multicenter, double-blind, randomized, placebo-controlled human cancer prevention trial in the December 25, 1996, issue of the *Journal of the American Medical Association* (Clark et al. 1996). In this study, 653 subjects received 200-microgram daily dietary selenium supplements and 659 subjects received placebos. Subjects receiving the selenium supplements had a 37% lower total cancer incidence, a 50% lower total cancer mortality, 45% fewer carcinomas, 63% fewer prostate cancers, 58% fewer colorectal cancers, and 46% fewer lung cancers than subjects in the placebo group.

The accumulated body of peer-reviewed scientific evidence supports the conclusion that dietary selenium supplementation by the at-risk population of Americans could prevent 480,000 new cancer cases each year, reducing the annual cancer expenditures by at least $12 billion.

So Why Doesn't Selenium Have the Support of the Medical Community?

If all the foregoing is true, it should raise some serious questions concerning the health care industry's apparent lack of interest in getting information presented to the public. This is fantastic news! Why hasn't everyone been told?

Of necessity, there must be some interval of time between important scientific discoveries and public awareness. In part, the delay is attributable to the fact that all scientific work must be verified by peer replication before it is generally accepted as fact. However, the requirement for validation can be abused, particularly if the acceptance of the data could have a substantial economic impact.

The probability of generating much interest and support from the medical community seems to be greater if the substance in question is a drug. Viewed from the perspective of financial incentive, this disparity is understandable. Drug status permits doctors to be paid for access to the substance and pharmaceutical companies to make substantial profits on the marketing of their products. To illustrate the point, physicians who appeared on television to comment upon research involving the drug tamoxifen described the substance as a "miracle" drug because it was shown to be useful for preventing as well as treating breast cancer. While much significance is attached to the fact that tamoxifen reduces breast cancer risk by about 50%, the fact that it was also found to more than double the risk of endometrial cancer seems to be of little importance. In contrast, research demonstrating that dietary selenium supplementation significantly reduces the incidence of several kinds of cancer in human populations with no reported evidence of associated toxicity, is described by members of the medical community as "potentially toxic" and "requires much additional study." While everyone would agree that more research would be desirable, time is critical for the current at-risk population that are middle-aged and above.

At present, there appears to be a conflict between the interest of the health care professionals and that of the general public. To the exact extent that we are successful in the prevention of any disease without employing drugs or vaccines, the demand for doctors, nurses, therapists, pharmacies and pharmaceutical companies, hospitals, medical supply companies, and all supporting personnel diminishes. In short, there is no financial incentive for the enthusiastic support of the use of dietary supplements.

Certainly, interest in disease prevention among the public is growing. In response to public pressures, medical schools have established new departments of preventive medicine and community health as well as new curricula, including nutrition. Hospitals and HMO's have opened "wellness centers," and food manufacturers are offering more and more low-fat or fat-free products. However encouraged we might be by the trends toward disease prevention, the real size of the commitment is measured by actual health care expenditures. In the case of cancer, for example, out of the $2.2 billion 1996 annual budget of the National Cancer Institute, only $200 million (less than 10%) is provided for prevention and control.

The United States Food and Drug Administration (FDA) makes clear distinctions between foods and drugs. Drugs must be proven safe and effective for specific disease treatments by passing the FDA drug protocol. While pharmaceutical companies may invest $200 million in satisfying the FDA protocol for a new drug, they can realize billions of dollars annually from the sale of a patented product. By contrast, the FDA regards food supplements as having no proven effects on diseases and, therefore, demonstrations of safety and effectiveness are not required. Moreover, food supplements cannot be protected by patent, so pharmaceutical companies cannot afford to invest their resources in either research or marketing of unprotected products.

Still another factor contributing to general ignorance of the health effects of dietary supplements is the sheer volume of scientific and medical research published each year. *Chemical Abstracts*, which lists authors, titles, and journals, along with brief summaries of published research papers, requires approximately twenty linear feet of library shelf space to accommodate the volumes citing the hundreds of thousands of research papers published each year. Just locating research papers on any given topic in the scientific literature is very time consuming. Considering that keeping abreast of medical research minimally requires a significant investment of time and that physicians work longer hours and have less free time than most people, it is unrealistic for us to expect our doctors to have a current, in-depth understanding of scientific research results on dietary supplements.

Reducing YOUR Cancer Risk

Although there is now general agreement that the proportions of carcinogens and anticarcinogens in our diets make up a significant part of our total cancer risk, it is unlikely that health care professionals, the Surgeon General, or government agencies will provide, in the immediate future, guidelines for reducing our cancer risk by the use of dietary supplements. No matter how extensive the data or how compelling the facts, there always appears to be a need for further research. Consider the comments of the National Research Council at the conclusion of their 1996 study of dietary carcinogens and anticarcinogens:

"Finally as advances are made in identifying with certainty certain specific naturally-occurring chemicals that either enhance or inhibit cancer risk in humans, it will be possible to formulate rational dietary guidelines for the American public." In the same issue of the *Journal of the American Medical Association* as Dr. Clark's impressive cancer prevention trial with dietary selenium, Dr. Graham A. Colditz wrote an editorial response entitled "Selenium and Cancer Prevention: Promising Results Indicate Further Trials Required" (Colditz 1996).

Eventually, the sheer weight of irrefutable scientific evidence will force even the most ardent conservatives to concede that specific dietary chemicals do, in fact, reduce our cancer risk when consumed in amounts greater than normally available in our diets. When that time finally arrives, such individuals will announce that only now are the data sufficiently conclusive to warrant using dietary supplements to reduce the risk of cancer.

Both history and personal experience tell us that many years will be required to convince the majority of Americans that many cancers can be avoided by appropriate changes in their diet. In the interim, our national cancer statistics are not likely to improve significantly.

The large number of Americans who are middle-aged or above must proactively pursue a lifestyle that can optimize their chances of enjoying many more cancer-free years. The most reliable source of sound information, free from economic bias, is the scientific literature. Unfortunately, most of us do not have either the time or the expertise to find and read with understanding the relevant studies. The purpose of this book is to present concisely the available scientific information on the singularly remarkable dietary anticarcinogen selenium so that everyone can make his or her own judgments about their dietary regimens. Citations are made to the primary scientific literature on each topic presented so that those interested can benefit from the insights of the physicians and scientists who conducted the original research.

CHAPTER 2

THE SELENIUM
—CANCER CONNECTION

"What can a man do who doesn't know what to do?"

—Milton Mayer

Naturally Occurring Selenium

Selenium enters the biosphere through volcanic activity. Consequently, the abundance of selenium in the environment depends upon the proximity of volcanoes where ash falling to the ground deposits selenium in soil. The West, particularly the Northwest, accounts for the volcanic deposition of selenium in the United States. Figure 2.1 shows those states affected by volcanic ashfall. The prevailing easterly winds carry ash to the Central Plains region of the United States so that the Mississippi River roughly constitutes the eastern-most extent of soils containing significant quantities of selenium. On the basis of soil selenium content alone, we might guess that people living in the Pacific Northwest would have the greatest amounts of selenium in the foods. As it turns out, soil selenium levels are only part of the story. Most of the selenium in volcanic ash will dissolve in water, so that in those geographic regions with large amounts of rain, the selenium quickly dissolves and combines with iron also leached from the soil. The new iron-selenium substances will not dissolve and are reincorporated into the soil. If the selenium is bound permanently in the soil, assimilation by plants and animals is virtually impossible. For example, Hawaii

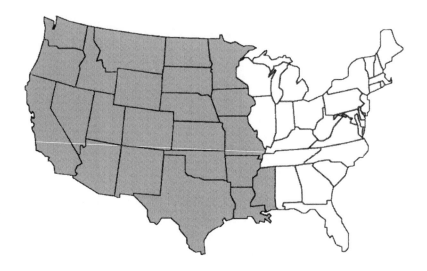

Fig. 2.1. States affected by volcanic ashfall

with its volcanoes has large amounts of soil selenium, but plants and animals living there contain very little selenium. The situation in Washington state and Oregon is similar to Hawaii—lots of volcanoes and selenium—but the plants and animals there tend to be selenium deficient. Thus, regions with volcanic ashfall and semiarid climates contain plants and animals with the greatest amounts of selenium. In 1967, J. Kubota and his associates (Kubota et al. 1967) published a paper describing the results of their measurements of selenium in alfalfa crops grown throughout the United States. Based upon alfalfa selenium levels, regions of the United States can be defined with higher, medium, and lower amounts of biologically available selenium. Figure 2.2 shows the distribution of selenium in alfalfa crops in the United States. With the knowledge that biologically available selenium depends upon volcanic ashfall **and** low annual rainfall, it is not surprising that the Central Plains region of the United States is the only place where both criteria are satisfied.

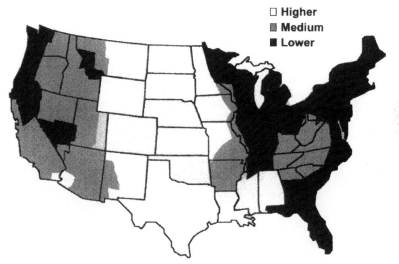

□ Higher
▨ Medium
■ Lower

Fig 2.2. Selenium levels in alfalfa

Archives of Environmental Health 46(1): 38, 1991. Reprinted with permission of the Helen Dwight Reid Educational Foundation, Published by Heldref Publications, 1319 Eighteenth St., Washington, DC 20036-1802.

Comparison of the distribution of selenium with that of population density in the United States leads to the disquieting realization that most people reside in regions with the lowest amounts of biologically-available selenium. The states in black in figure 2.3 collectively account for 73% of the total population. There is, indeed, a striking correspondence of the United States population centers in figure 2.3 with the lower selenium (black) regions shown in figure 2.2.

Discovery of the Selenium —Human Cancer Relationship

As early as 1976, Shamberger and his colleagues (Shamberger, Tytko, and Willis 1976) published their work in which the United States was divided into high-, medium-, and low-selenium states according to the alfalfa data of Kubota. Their data showed that cancer death rates increased as biologically-available selenium decreased with a statistical confidence of 99.9% (meaning that there is only one chance in a thousand that these results could have occurred by chance alone). These investigators also reported that

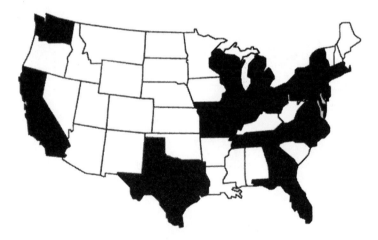

Fig. 2.3. States collectively comprising 73% of the United States population

cancer death rates among residents in 19 cities of the United States decreased as average blood selenium levels in those cities increased with a statistical confidence of 95%.

The findings of Shamberger's research group were corroborated independently by others (Cowgill 1983) and (Clark, Cantor, and Allaway 1991). As with all generally-accepted scientific work, the high-selenium-low-cancer relationship was validated by replication. These epidemiological studies **strongly suggest** but **do not prove** that people living in areas with small amounts of biologically-available selenium in the United States have a greater risk of developing cancer.

Selenium-Cancer Studies in Other Countries

If the selenium-cancer risk relationship observed in the United States is real, then one would expect the same relationship to be found in other countries of the world as well. In 1977, G. N. Schrauzer's research group (Schrauzer, White, and Schneider 1977) published the results of their study of the relationships between dietary and blood levels of seven minerals, including selenium, and cancer deaths occurring in 28 countries of the world. These investigators found that countries with higher per capita dietary selenium intakes or higher blood levels of selenium had significantly lower death rates from leukemia and cancers of the intestine, rectum, prostate, breast, ovary, lung, pancreas, skin, and bladder.

China is especially interesting to those studying the relationships between diet and disease because food is grown and consumed in the same geographic area. Consequently, diseases that are more prevalent in any given region can be attributed to the amount of a particular food component unique to the people of that specific region. In 1985, a study of cancer death rates and blood selenium levels in 24 regions distributed among eight provinces in China was reported (Yu et al. 1985). As with previous studies, Yu and colleagues found that regions with high blood selenium levels had lower cancer death rates.

These investigators also conducted a particularly interesting study in 43 communes in Qidong County of Jiangsu Province. As it happens, Qidong

County is one of the high-risk areas for liver cancer in China, with higher incidences of liver cancer in the southern part of the county than in the north. Selenium analysis of the corn and maize throughout the county revealed that selenium levels in these crops were lowest in the southern part of the county, where liver cancer incidence was significantly higher.

As in North America and Asia, cancer incidence was related to biologically-available selenium in Europe as well. J. T. Salonen and his research associates (Salonen et al. 1984) measured blood selenium levels in approximately 8,000 cancer-free men and women living in eastern Finland and monitored the cancer deaths in these individuals over a period of five years. By the sixth year of the study, 85 additional people had developed cancer. For each person who either developed or died of cancer, a cancer-free cohort matched as closely as possible for sex, age, number of cigarettes smoked per day, etc. was chosen for comparison. Blood selenium levels of cancer patients (measured before they developed cancer) were significantly lower than their cancer-free cohorts with a statistical confidence of 98.8%.

One Finnish study (P. Knekt et al. 1998) is particularly interesting because it demonstrated that higher blood (serum) levels of selenium were associated with a reduction in lung cancer risk in nonsmokers and an even greater reduction in smokers. Blood samples from 9,101 cancer-free subjects were obtained during the 1968-1971 and 1973-1976 time periods. By 1991, 95 subjects had developed lung cancer. 190 cancer-free subjects matched for age, gender, and place of residence were selected for comparison. Nonsmokers with serum selenium levels in the highest third of measured samples had a 59% lower cancer risk than those with serum selenium levels in the lowest third of measured values. Impressively, smokers with serum selenium levels in the highest third of measured values had an 84% lower lung cancer risk than those with blood selenium values in the lowest third of measured samples.

The satisfying aspect of all these studies is their consistency. They all show that greater amounts of selenium in humans are invariably associated with lower cancer incidence at a comfortably high level of confidence.

More Good News

If greater dietary quantities of selenium can protect humans from cancer, it should also be possible to demonstrate that comparable amounts (based upon body weight) also protect laboratory animals from cancer. Happily, there are literally scores of studies confirming precisely that. Without describing in bone-crushing detail each of these studies, I want you to be informed sufficiently that you have no lingering doubts about the anticarcinogenic effectiveness of selenium taken in nontoxic doses.

Schrauzer and Ishmael conducted a study in which a particular strain of mouse (C_3H/St) was chosen because 80-95% of these inbred animals develop spontaneous breast cancers (Schrauzer and Ishmael 1974). One group of mice was given selenium in their drinking water and another group was given none. In the group receiving no selenium in their water, 22 out of 30 mice (82%) ultimately developed breast cancer. By comparison, only three out of 30 animals (10%) given selenium in their drinking water developed breast cancer.

In a similar study, Dr. Clement Ip used the carcinogen dimethylbenzanthracene (DMBA) to produce breast cancers in a particular strain of rats eating diets with differing amounts of fat (Ip 1983). Without selenium supplementation, 40% of rats eating a low-fat (5%) diet developed breast cancer from the DMBA, while 70% of those on high-fat (25%) diet suffered DMBA-induced breast cancer. When diets were supplemented with selenium, rats on the low-fat diet experienced a 16% reduction in the incidence of DMBA-induced breast cancers and the animals on the high-fat diet had a 25% breast cancer reduction. These findings support two important conclusions:

1. Animals on high-fat diets have a greater cancer risk.
2. Dietary selenium supplements produce greater cancer risk reduction in animals on high-fat diets.

Drs. Medina and Lane also used DMBA to induce breast cancers in mice that normally have a very low incidence of such cancers (Medina and Lane 1983). They found that DMBA exposure produced breast cancers in 56% of unsupplemented mice compared to only 16% in the animals receiving a dietary selenium supplement.

Although the studies sketched above constitute a very small fraction of the animal data, they are representative of the typical result of these types of investigation. The real strength of this body of data is its consistency. All studies using naturally-occurring chemical forms of selenium show some degree of protection from cancer. Obviously, it is more satisfying to study the effects of selenium upon human cancers.

Human Cancer Cells

The effects of selenium upon human cancer cells also can be studied *in vitro* (meaning in an artificial environment). Cancer cells that have been surgically removed from patients can be grown in the laboratory. Unlike normal cells, cancer cells are immortal (divide indefinitely). Consequently, cancer cell cultures can be maintained for many years and are most useful in evaluating substances to be used for cancer prevention and chemotherapy.

Watrach and his research group (Watrach et al. 1984) studied the effects of selenium upon two human breast cancer cell lines identified as MCF-7 and MDA-MB-231 and a normal human embryonal lung cell line MCR-5. Three days after the addition of 0.42 micrograms of selenium to each milliliter of the three separate cell cultures, examination of the cultures revealed that the selenium had killed 55% of the MCF-7 cancer cells and 45% of the MDA-MB-231 cancer cells, while 100% of the non-malignant lung cells remained alive. This experiment demonstrates that selenium can kill human cancer cells at dose levels that are non-toxic to healthy human cells. It is especially exciting to realize that the selenium levels that killed a significant fraction of the cancer cells in this study were the same as actual blood levels in humans living in high-selenium geographic areas (Longnecker et al. 1991).

The Ultimate Test

Even with two decades of epidemiological, laboratory animal, and *in vitro* cancer cell evidence that selenium can reduce the risk of cancer, no one had actually given healthy human research subjects dietary selenium supplements under carefully controlled guidelines to determine whether or not such supplementation could prevent them from developing cancer. In 1983, Dr. Larry C. Clark at the Arizona Cancer Center and others at Cornell University along with participating physicians at seven dermatology clinics in the eastern United States (Clark et al. 1996) began their double-blind, placebo-controlled cancer-prevention trial. During the period from 1983 to 1991, patients with histories of basal cell or squamous cell carcinomas were recruited and randomly assigned to receive either a 200-microgram selenium supplement or a placebo. In all, 1,312 patients with an average age of 63 were included in the study. The original objective was to determine whether or not dietary selenium supplements could reduce the incidence of non-melanoma skin cancers. Surprisingly, selenium supplements had no effect on the incidence of skin cancers, but produced dramatic reductions in prostate, lung, and colorectal cancers. In 1990, the objectives of the study were broadened to include the effects of selenium supplements on total mortality and cancer mortality, in addition to the incidences of lung, colorectal, and prostate cancers. The interim results of the study were sufficiently impressive that the Safety Monitoring and Advisory Committee recommended that the study be terminated and the findings published upon completion of the tenth year. The statistically-significant percentage risk reductions in the several categories of cancer achieved by subjects with dietary selenium supplementation compared to subjects taking placebos were: total cancer 37%, total cancer mortality 50%, total carcinomas 45%, prostate cancers 63%, colorectal cancers 58%, lung cancers 46%, and lung cancer mortality 53%.

Concurrent with Dr. Clark's study in the United States, four other cancer prevention trials in humans using selenium supplementation were conducted in China. In 1991, S.-Y. Yu and his research team (Yu et al. 1991) published the results of two separate trials involving research subjects living in Qidong County. Both trials were designed to establish whether or not dietary selenium supplementation could reduce the incidence of primary liver cancer, which occurs with notoriously-high incidence in this geographic area. One trial involved five townships with approximate populations varying from 20,000 to 32,000 and having essentially identical incidences of liver cancer. One township of approximately 20,000 individuals was provided with table salt containing 0.00056% selenium, while the remaining four townships, with a collective population of some 110,000 using selenium-free salt, served as a comparison group. During the five-year trial (1985-1990), the township using the selenium-enriched salt experienced 43% fewer incidences of liver cancer compared to the townships using selenium-free salt.

In a second, two-year trial (Yu et al. 1991), 200-microgram dietary selenium supplements or a placebo were given randomly to 2,474 persons whose families were subject to a higher incidence of liver cancer. In all, 1,444 received selenium supplements, while 1,030 were given placebos for comparison. Liver cancer incidence in the selenium-supplemented subjects was reduced by 45% compared to the placebo group with a statistical confidence of 95%. Although neither trial was conducted using a double-blind protocol, the findings of these trials are remarkably similar to those of Dr. Clark's study in the United States.

A third Chinese trial (Blot et al. 1993) was conducted in the period from 1986 to 1991 and involved the administration of various vitamin/mineral supplements to 29,584 research subjects from four Linxian communes. Subjects were divided into four groups receiving either vitamin A and zinc, or riboflavin and niacin, or vitamin C and molybdenum, or β-carotene, selenium, and vitamin E. The only group with a statistically-significant reduction in cancer mortality was the group receiving the β-carotene, selenium, and vitamin E supplement. In this group, total cancer mortality decreased by 13% and mortality from stomach cancer decreased by 21% with a statistical confidence of 95%.

The 13% reduction in total cancer mortality found in the Linxian trial is much less impressive than either the Qidong or United States trials. Most likely the explanation is related to the size of the selenium supplements used. In the Linxian study only 50-microgram supplements were used, compared to the 200-microgram supplements employed in both the Qidong and U.S. trials. The proportionally greater protection achieved in the United States and Qidong trials emphasizes the importance of supplementing with an appropriately-large dose of selenium.

The fourth Chinese trial conducted by J-Y. Li and colleagues (Li et al. 1993) in the same time period (1985-1991) produced very different results from the United States trial and the other three Chinese trials and illustrates still another interesting and important aspect of nutritional supplementation. In this trial 3,318 subjects with pre-malignant esophageal cells were assigned randomly to receive either a supplement containing 26 vitamins and minerals or a placebo. No statistically-significant differences in cancer mortality between the supplementation and placebo groups were found. The scientists conducting this trial were apparently unaware of both animal (Schrauzer, White and Schneider 1976) and epidemiological (Schrauzer, White, and Schneider 1977) studies providing evidence that zinc, taken in sufficiently large amounts, can abolish the cancer protection afforded by selenium. In a later chapter, I shall explain how zinc's interference with selenium's ability to prevent cancer is accounted for by understanding the manner in which selenium exerts its anticarcinogenic benefit.

It is important to appreciate that cancer-prevention trials involving thousands of research subjects demonstrate that dietary selenium supplementation is effective at nontoxic dose levels. Although not required by statute, it is satisfying to know that scientists throughout the world are establishing that dietary selenium supplementation is safe and effective without the supervision of the United States Food and Drug Administration.

Selenium's Importance to You

Considering the terrible suffering, expense, and mortality inflicted by cancer, it would seem irrational not to do anything that could lessen your risk of developing the disease—particularly if it can been done safely without completely overhauling your lifestyle. Those of us middle-aged or above are at risk for cancer. All the existing data indicate dietary selenium supplementation could be a powerful weapon in our cancer prevention arsenal.

Your decision whether or not to supplement your dietary selenium should be based upon as complete an understanding of the relevant facts as possible. Is there more than one kind of naturally-occurring selenium? What do our bodies do with selenium? How docs selenium prevent cancer? What amount of selenium is safe and effective? Is too much selenium toxic? What are the symptoms of selenium toxicity? Do other dietary components interfere with or potentiate selenium's ability to prevent cancer? Are all commercially available selenium supplements equivalent? The following chapters provide you with the facts you'll need to make a more informed decision.

CHAPTER 3

CRITICAL DIFFERENCES IN NATURAL SELENIUM

"The scientist takes off from the manifold observations of predecessors and shows his intelligence, if any, by his ability to discriminate between the important and the negligible, by selecting here and there the significant stepping stones that will lead across difficulties to new understanding."

Hans Zinsser

Is All Selenium Created Equal?

Dramatic differences in cancer prevention afforded by the several chemical forms of naturally-occurring dietary selenium make it important for us to understand the reasons for these crucial differences. It is axiomatic that anyone considering dietary selenium supplementation for cancer prevention would choose the naturally-occurring chemical form with the greatest prophylactic benefit. Such differences are obvious in the laboratory, consistent from one study to another, and make perfect sense in terms of the different human metabolic pathways imposed upon the several chemical forms. The importance of educating ourselves about various forms of dietary selenium becomes evident when we realize that commercially-available dietary selenium supplements sold in the United States contain different chemical forms of selenium and, consequently, may differ in their cancer-preventive effectiveness. Lacking the relevant information, we cannot reliably choose the most effective supplement.

A word of advice: don't be intimidated by the funny names of the various chemical forms of selenium. They are just used for identification.

The Chemical forms of Naturally-Occurring Selenium

Selenium present in volcanic ash enters the biosphere in three chemical forms: elemental selenium, hydrogen selenide, and selenium dioxide. Upon contact with natural water, selenium is converted into two additional forms called selenite and selenate. These five environmental forms are mineral forms and are referred to as inorganic selenium. Figure 3.1 shows the structural formulas of the inorganic forms of selenium. Plants and animals convert inorganic selenium into the organic forms they need. The most

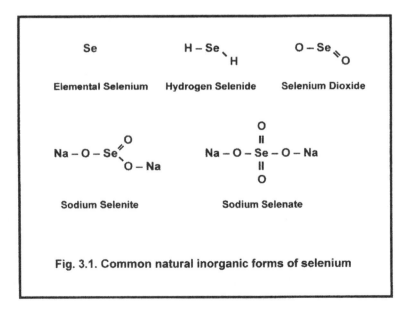

Fig. 3.1. Common natural inorganic forms of selenium

abundant organic forms of selenium found in organisms are the amino acids used for making proteins. The most common and, therefore, the most studied selenium-containing amino acids are selenomethionine, selenocysteine, and methlyselenocysteine. Structures of these three important selenium-containing amino acids are shown in figure 3.2.

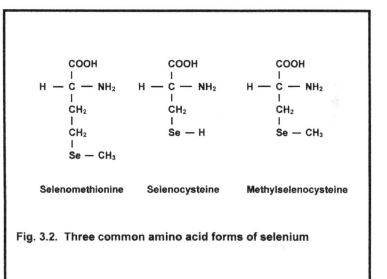

Selenomethionine   **Selenocysteine**   **Methylselenocysteine**

Fig. 3.2. Three common amino acid forms of selenium

For the most part, inorganic (mineral) forms of selenium such as selenite and selenate are found in natural water. With the exception of a few isolated communities having substantial quantities of inorganic selenium in their drinking water, most people derive their dietary selenium from their food in one of the several amino acid (organic) forms. In these compounds (forms) selenium (Se) is taking a place more typically occupied by sulfur. Selenomethionine is perhaps the most common selenoamino acid constituting approximately 50% of the selenium in wheat (Olsen et al. 1970) and about 85%of the selenium in high-selenium yeast (Ip et al. 2000). In the same study, methylselenocysteine was found to comprise some 73% of the selenium in high-selenium garlic. Other investigators have reported that methylselenocysteine is also one of the forms present in high-selenium yeast (Bird et al.1997).

What Our Bodies Do with Dietary Selenium

Regardless of the chemical form of selenium consumed in the diet, it is ultimately modified chemically (metabolized) to make the form essential to our cells. Human cells make a dozen or so proteins called selenoproteins that contain selenium in the form of selenocysteine (Ip and Hayes 1989). From a nutritional point of view, all dietary selenium is used to make selenocysteine, which is strategically incorporated in the important selenoproteins essential to our cells. Selenoproteins are enzymes and, therefore, have unique responsibilities in the cell. Since enzymes are recycled, selenoproteins are needed only in small amounts, and cellular levels are carefully regulated. Dietary selenium in excess of that needed to make selenoproteins is converted to chemical forms suitable for excretion.

In human cells, hydrogen selenide is the starting place for making selenoproteins so that dietary selenium must first be converted to hydrogen selenide (Sunde 1984). The series of forms produced from ingestion to excretion is called the metabolic pathway and differs for the various inorganic and organic forms. Such differences account for the non-trivial disparity in anticarcinogenic activity consistently seen between the several forms of dietary selenium. Figure 3.3 shows the metabolic pathway for inorganic selenium. Two of the forms produced metabolically (metabolites)—selenodiglutathione and

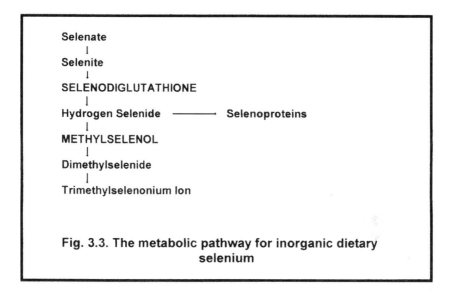

Fig. 3.3. The metabolic pathway for inorganic dietary selenium

methylselenol—are represented in capital letters because they play key roles in selenium's anticarcinogenic activity. Both selenodiglutatione (Milner and Fico 1987) and methylselenol (Vanhanavikit, Ip, and Ganther 1993) are considered to be among the most potent known selenium anticarcinogens. Selenodiglutathione kills cancer cells so effectively that its sterile solutions have been patented for direct injection into cancers. Notice that selenodiglutathione is the very first metabolite produced when selenite is the dietary form of selenium. Since all human cells contain glutathione, selenite combines with cellular glutathione to produce selenodiglutathione.

Organic forms of dietary selenium also produce methylselenol, but not selenodiglutathione. On this basis, one might guess *a priori* that organic forms of dietary selenium might be less effective in preventing cancer than selenite. As it happens, most organic forms of dietary selenium are, indeed, less effective anticarcinogens than selenite. Only those organic forms producing methylselenol as their first metabolite are known to compete effectively (Ganther 1999). Methylselenocysteine, the major selenium-containing constituent in high-selenium garlic (Cai et al. 1995), is the only selenoaminoacid that produces sufficiently high levels of methylselenol to be an excellent anticarcinogen (as good as selenite). The metabolic pathway for methylselenocysteine is shown in figure 3.4. The initial metabolite of methylselenocysteine is methylselenol, one of the two most potent known selenium anticarcinogens.

Methylselenocysteine
  |
METHYLSELENOL — Hydrogen Selenide — Selenoproteins
  |
Dimethylselenide
  |
Trimethylselenonium Ion

Fig. 3.4. The metabolic pathway for methylselenocysteine

If we compare the metabolic pathway for selenomethionine and selenocysteine, the two most common organic forms of naturally-occurring dietary selenium, with that of methylselenocysteine, the reason for the anticarcinogenic superiority of methylselenocysteine is apparent. Figure 3.5 illustrates the metabolic pathway for selenomethionine and selenocysteine. In the case of selenocysteine, the first metabolic product is not one of the two most potent selenium anticarcinogens. The explanation for the relative ineffectiveness of selenomethionine in preventing cancer is its removal from the metabolic pool by insertion into body proteins. Here it is important to understand that the DNA in our cells can distinguish between cysteine, a sulfur containing amino acid, and selenocysteine that is identical to cysteine except the sulfur in cysteine is replaced with selenium. This discriminating ability guarantees that selenocysteines are accurately placed in all of the essential selenoprotein enzymes. On the other hand, our cellular DNA cannot distinguish between the sulfur-containing methionine and its selenium-containing analog selenomethionine. The result is that selenomethionine is randomly inserted into body proteins in place of methionine. Once the selenomethionine is incorporated into a protein, it becomes biologically inactive and cannot generate either of the two potent selenium anticarcinogens. In fact, many proteins such as hair, nails, skin, etc. are either cut or sloughed off so that selenomethionine present in these tissues is excreted. Among the various forms of naturally-occurring dietary selenium, selenomethionine is unique in that it produces very high tissue levels of selenium (Ip 1998).

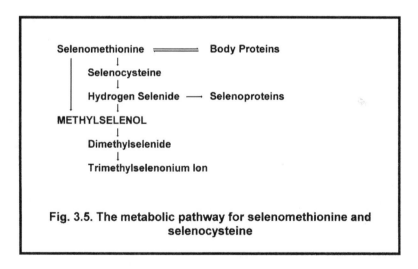

Fig. 3.5. The metabolic pathway for selenomethionine and selenocysteine

The cancer-prevention consequences of storing a portion of dietary selenium in proteins was demonstrated by Dr. Clement Ip and his research group (Ip and Hayes 1989). These researchers divided female rats into three groups. One group was given a dietary selenium supplement in the form of selenite, and a second group was given the same amount of selenium in the form of selenomethionine. A control group received no selenium supplement. Breast cancers were induced in the three groups with identical doses of the carcinogen dimethylbenzanthracene to compare the cancer protection afforded by inorganic and organic selenium supplements. Selenium levels were measured in blood, liver, kidney, and skeletal muscle of rats from both the selenite and selenomethionine groups to compare the amount of selenium stored in tissue proteins. Rats given selenomethionine were found to have higher selenium levels in all tissues. The selenomethionine-supplemented rats with high tissue levels of selenium, however, inhibited breast cancer incidence by only 45% compared to 73% inhibition in the selenite-supplemented rats. Obviously, the amount of selenium stored in tissues is unrelated to protection from cancer. Unfortunately, the fact that selenomethionine-containing supplements produce higher tissue selenium levels has been used to suggest that selenomethionine is absorbed more readily than other forms of dietary selenium. This is not true. In fact, a 1976 study (Whanger et al. 1976) demonstrated that selenite and selenomethionine were absorbed to the same extent from the digestive tracts of rats. In addition, an evaluation of commercially-available high-selenium yeast found no difference between the absorption of selenite and high-selenium yeast (Spallholz and Raferty 1987). If our objectives are to reduce our cancer risk and provide our bodies with the selenium they need for making essential selenoproteins, then taking dietary selenium in the form of selenomethionine is much less effective.

The clear superiority of selenite over most forms of organic selenium has been demonstrated repeatedly in animal studies. In 1980, Drs. Greeder and Milner published their study comparing the anticarcinogenic effectiveness of three inorganic forms of selenium with that of selenomethionine and selenocystine (Greeder and Milner 1980). They divided laboratory mice into six groups. One group was given no selenium supplement; the other five groups were given equivalent amounts of selenium in the forms of selenium dioxide, sodium selenite, sodium selenate, selenomethionine, or selenocystine. All six groups were injected with 500,000 live Ehrlich ascites tumor cells. None of the mice receiving the three inorganic forms of selenium developed ascites tumors. In sharp contrast, 100% of the unsupplemented mice, 100% of the selenomethionine-supplemented mice, and 40% of the selenocystine-supplemented mice developed ascites tumors. The superior anticarcinogenic activity of selenite relative to selenomethionine was also demonstrated by Dr. Henry Thompson (Thompson 1984) and by Dr. A. C. Griffin (Griffin and Jacobs 1977).

Before we leave the subject of metabolic pathways for the various chemical forms of dietary selenium, I want to call your attention to two important features common to all pathways. First, the dietary forms of selenium actually ingested are not the best anticarcinogens. Indeed, the two most potent anticarcinogens—selenodiglutathione and methylselenol—are intermediate metabolites produced in the metabolism of dietary forms. Consequently, the only times these more effective anticarcinogens are produced are those times when our bodies are actively modifying dietary selenium. Appreciating this fact makes us aware of the importance of supplementing our selenium continuously. Second, methylselenol does not accumulate in significant amounts until after the selenoproteins have reached their controlled levels. When selenium in excess of that needed to make selenoproteins is ingested, the excess is converted into forms suitable for excretion. Excess selenium is initially converted into methylselenol for excretion in the urine. When larger amounts are taken, some of the excess is converted to dimethylselenide that is exhaled in the lungs. With still larger amounts are ingested, a third excretory metabolite trimethylselenonium ion is produced for urinary excretion (Ganther 1986). Thus, it is apparent that larger amounts of the important anticarcinogen methylselenol are not generated until **excess** selenium is taken (Combs 1999). Ingesting more selenium than we need nutritionally (called a supranutritional amount) is very important to reducing our cancer risk.

Using Your Knowledge of Selenium

From an application point of view, our understanding of selenium metabolism should focus our attention on three important ideas:

1. dietary forms of selenium that produce either selenodiglutathione or methylselenol as their first metabolites are more effective than any other forms of selenium;

2. the two most effective known selenium anticarcinogens are produced only during the active metabolism of dietary forms so that continuous daily supplementation provides the greatest cancer-prevention benefit;

3. dietary selenium in excess of that needed to make selenoproteins must be taken to produce significant amounts of the excellent anticarcinogen methylselenol.

Many questions essential to intelligent selenium supplementation remain. How much selenium should be added to the selenium I am already getting in my diet? Is too much selenium toxic? How much is too much? What are the signs of selenium toxicity? Are there other vitamins and minerals that interfere with or enhance selenium's ability to prevent cancer? What selenium supplements are available commercially, and how do I know which chemical forms they contain? The following chapters will give you insights into these and other issues.

CHAPTER 4

SELENIUM-INDUCED CANCER CELL SUICIDE

*"Truth can never be told so as to be understood
and not be believed."*

William Blake

Introduction

In Chapter 3 we learned that naturally-occurring dietary selenium is distributed among several chemical forms differing substantially in their ability to prevent cancer. In the present chapter we shall again consult the scientific and medical research literature for answers to questions about how cells become malignant and the role selenium plays in cancer prevention. That selenium is an effective anticarcinogen and that dietary selenium supplementation can substantially reduce the incidence of cancer in humans are now scientific facts. The goals of the present cancer-related selenium research are to understand precisely how selenium exerts its cancer-protection benefit and to determine the specific chemical form that is most effective and, at the same time, the least toxic. Understanding the differences in the mechanisms by which the several chemical forms of dietary selenium inhibit the initiation and promotion of cancer is important in choosing a selenium supplement.

Oxygen-Induced Cell Damage —Normal Wear and Tear

With the help of certain proteins called enzymes, our cells use the oxygen we inhale to literally burn the food we eat for the energy we need to live. The oxygen we inhale is converted in a series of steps from oxygen to superoxide ion, to hydrogen peroxide, to hydroxyl radical, and ultimately, to water. The three forms of oxygen generated between oxygen gas and water are high-energy (very chemically active) substances that can alter (damage) most substances they encounter. These species are toxic to cells, so that cells must have antioxidants to keep oxygen-associated damage to a minimum. Interestingly, some white blood cells called phagocytes (cell-eating cells) deliberately produce chemically active oxygen species precisely for the purpose of killing unwanted cells. If a bacterium infects our bodies, a phagocyte may engulf the invading bacterial cell, releasing a burst of superoxide and hydrogen peroxide to kill the bacterium. Antioxidants are substances that combine readily with active oxygen species. The presence of ample amounts of antioxidants makes it more likely that active oxygen species will be consumed before they have an opportunity to damage critical cell components.

If chemically active oxygen species happen to damage cellular DNA, the consequences can be serious. Instructions for making each essential protein in a cell are located in segments of DNA called genes. If a particular gene is damaged, the protein it encodes is either made incorrectly or not at all, and the cell is said to be mutated. Substances capable of damaging cellular DNA are referred to as genotoxic. When mutated cells encounter carcinogens, the cell can become transformed into a cancer cell.

How Human Cells Become Malignant

The transformation from normal to cancerous cells is a two-step process. The steps are called initiation and promotion. Initiation occurs when the DNA of cells is damaged by high-energy radiation (e.g. X-rays or UV light), reactive forms of oxygen, carcinogens, or errors in DNA replication for cell division. Cells with damaged DNA are sometimes called mutated cells or pre-cancerous cells. Exposure of pre-cancerous cells to tumor promoters results in the promotion step. Tumor promoters are substances that activate cancer-producing genes (proto-oncogenes) or deactivate tumor-suppressor genes. Activation of proto-oncogenes produces oncogenes, which cause cells to undergo unregulated proliferation. Tumor-suppressor genes, on the other hand, are those that actively regulate cell reproduction. Cells than have undergone both initiation and promotion are called transformed (malignant) cells. Whether or not malignant cells develop into clinically detectable cancers depends upon how fast the cells die.

Cell Death—Murder and Suicide

In order for humans to remain healthy, there must be some way to get rid of cells that are old, no longer needed, or dangerous. Skin cells damaged by the sun or GI tract cells damaged by carcinogens in our food could become malignant if there were no mechanism for their disposal. Although we are unaware of it, over **3,000,000,000** cells in our bodies die **every minute.** Such cells must die either by necrosis or apoptosis.

Necrosis is a more traumatic cell death caused by external factors that essentially murder the cell. Physical or chemical insult, heat, oxygen deficiency, or loss of blood supply can result in necrosis. Necrotic cells can no longer control water entry so they swell and rupture, spilling cellular material into surrounding tissues and triggering an inflammatory response from the immune system.

Apoptosis, however, is an internally (genetically) programmed cell suicide. In multi-cellular organisms, apoptosis seems to be an altruistic suicide committed by defective cells that preserves the life of the organism and allows the remaining healthy cells to perpetuate their undamaged genes. Apoptosis can be triggered by chemical signals from other cells or genetic (DNA) damage caused by high-energy radiation, virus infection, old age, heat, or anticancer drugs. Even though all cells contain suicide genes, it is important to realize that apoptosis does not occur randomly and is limited to problem cells. Conditions that initiate suicide in problem cells are insufficient to produce apoptosis in normal cells. Cells that are especially susceptible to apoptotic triggers are called primed cells. The unregulated proliferation of cancer cells does not initiate apoptosis but greatly enhances their responses to apoptotic triggers.

Virtually all of the 3,000,000,000 cells that die in our bodies each minute are undergoing apoptosis. We are not aware of this mass suicide because apoptosis is a quiet, natural form of cell death. Apoptotic cells shrink away from their neighbors, cut up their DNA, package the DNA fragments and cellular organelles in cell membrane, and the resulting packages (apoptotic bodies) are consumed by other cells. There is no inflammatory response because the cell parts are cleverly wrapped in membranes.

How Cells Commit Suicide

Apoptosis can be triggered by biological agents that alter the cell's reproductive cycle. Inhibition of the enzymes that regulate the cell cycle leads to arrests in one of the cell-cycle checkpoints and, subsequently, to apoptosis. The protein kinase C (PKC) enzyme family exerts anti-apoptotic effects that mediate cell survival. Inhibition of PKC has been shown to initiate apoptosis in a variety of cancer cells (Jarvis and Grant 1999). For example, the two PKC inhibitors tamoxifen and staurosporine have been shown (McCarty 1998) to induce apoptosis in human malignant glioma and Burkitt's lymphoma cells.

Cell-cycle arrest and apoptosis also can be induced by agents that damage DNA (genotoxic agents). Among the 100,000 or so genes in the DNA of our cells are those that can cause cell suicide when activated in response to some apoptotic trigger such as DNA damage. One such gene is called p53. The "p" stands for the protein it produces, and the "53" indicates the size of the protein. In normal cells the protein produced by the p53 gene survives for a very short time (about 20 minutes), but in damaged cells the protein remains. The presence of the p53 protein causes, among other things, the cell's reproductive cycle to be arrested in either the G_1 or the G_2/M or the G_0-G_1-S checkpoints (Levine 1997). During cell-cycle arrest, DNA is repaired, or apoptosis is initiated when DNA damage is too severe for repair. In effect, the p53 gene is responsible for maintaining the integrity of genetic information in the cell.

If the p53 gene itself is damaged by some mutagenic agent, the cell can proceed to S phase (the reproductive phase), resulting in cell division. Cells with mutated p53 genes allow damaged cells to proliferate and increase the risk of cancer. In fact, an estimated 70% of human cancers have inoperative p53 genes (McCarthy, Herrington, and Evan 1996). Damage protection of cellular DNA by p53 is so effective that some viruses have developed the ability to deactivate p53 as a strategy for efficient viral reproduction (Sarnow et al. 1982). Since viruses insert their DNA into that of the infected cell in order to reproduce, p53 presents a problem. Inserted viral DNA is interpreted as genetic damage, and p53 initiates apoptosis. Viral reproduction depends upon the host cell remaining alive and inactivation of the p53 gene prevents the host cell from committing suicide.

Whether apoptosis is triggered by inhibition of cell-cycle enzymes or by DNA damage, all cells execute apoptosis using the same cell-suicide machinery. Cell death is dependent upon cutting the cell's double-stranded DNA into small pieces by a calcium/magnesium-dependent endonuclease enzyme. Consequently, the minerals calcium and magnesium as well as the endonuclease are all essential components of the cell's suicide machinery. The endonuclease cannot do its cutting job without the assistance of both calcium (Ca^{+2}) and magnesium (Mg^{+2}). In fact, anything that interferes with the participation of either calcium or magnesium can prevent apoptosis from occurring and, thereby, increases the risk of cancer. Because it is known that the mineral zinc (Zn) interferes with endonuclease activity (Tanuma 1996), these researchers could demonstrate that the Ca/Mg-dependent endonuclease was doing the cutting by preventing apoptosis with the addition of zinc. Zinc interference with endonuclease activity is the most likely explanation for Dr. Schrauzer's much earlier (Schrauzer, White, and Schneider 1976) demonstration that dietary zinc supplementation can abolish the cancer prevention effectiveness of selenium supplements. Since calcium is essential for endonuclease activity and, thus, cell suicide, you will not be surprised to learn that hypertension drugs that reduce cellular calcium (calcium channel blockers) also interfere with apoptosis and increase the risk of several different cancers (Pahor et al. 1996).

Apoptosis and Cancer

Research conducted in the last two decades has led to the conclusion that apoptosis plays a critical role in cancer promotion (Harmon and Allen 1996). The progression or remission of cancer depends upon the relative rates of cell proliferation and apoptosis (Schulte-Hermann et al. 1995). Although cancer cells have elevated rates of proliferation, they also have increased rates of apoptosis. In those instances where apoptotic rates exceed rates of proliferation, the cancer may disappear altogether (Schulte-Hermann 1990). Studies to date suggest that cancer progression results from tumor promoters causing a decrease in the rate of apoptosis (Tomei, Kantor, and Wenner 1988). Thus, cancer progression is more dependent upon the reduction of the apoptotic rate than the acceleration of cell division.

Selenium and Cancer Cell Suicide

The overwhelming majority of existing evidence supports the conclusion that selenium exerts most of its anticarcinogenic effects by inducing apoptosis in premalignant and malignant cells. The significant differences consistently seen between the anticarcinogenic effectiveness of the several naturally-occurring chemical forms of selenium suggest that the biochemical mechanisms involved in the antitumor activity of the various chemical forms must be fundamentally distinct. The three most abundant known naturally-occurring chemical forms of selenium—selenomethionine, methylselenocysteine , and selenite—have been more intensively investigated and differ in their antitumor mechanisms and effectiveness.

Selenite-Induced Apoptosis in Cancer Cells

As early as 1994 selenodiglutathione, the initial metabolite of selenite, was reported (Lanfear et al. 1994) to induce apoptosis in both human ovarian A2780 cancer cells with unmutated (wild-type) p53 and in mouse erytroleukemia (MEL) cells with mutated p53 genes. These investigators demonstrated that the addition of either selenodiglutathione or cisplatin, a widely-used chemotherapeutic agent, induced the overexpression of the p53 protein and apoptosis in the ovarian cancer cells with wild-type p53. These findings indicated that both selenodiglutathione and cisplatin were causing DNA damage in the ovarian cancer cells and, thereby, were inducing apoptosis by the p53-mediated damage recognition pathway.

Interestingly, the MEL cells with mutated (inactive) p53 were also very effectively killed by selenodiglutathione. This finding demonstrated that the selenodiglutathione induction of apoptosis in cancer cells is not solely dependent upon p53. Selenite, methylselenocysteine, and dimethyl selenoxide also inhibited the growth of both A2760 and MEL cells, but less effectively than selenodiglutathione. The addition of glutathione enhanced the antitumor effectiveness of selenite, indicating that selenite and glutathione were reacting to produce the more effective selenodiglutathione.

The early evidence that the anticarcinogenic effects of selenium are attributable to the induction of apoptosis prompted a 1996 study (Zhu et al. 1996) using A172 and T98G human brain cancer cell lines and non-malignant NT14 fibroblast cells. The chemical form of selenium chosen for the study was sodium selenite. The addition of equal amounts of selenium to the three cell cultures resulted in the induction of apoptosis in the two cancer cell lines, but was without effect on the non-malignant fibroblast cells. The selenium-induced apoptosis in the cancer cell lines could be prevented by the addition of catalase, which is known to react chemically with reactive oxygen species. These finding prompted the authors to conclude that the cancer cell apoptosis was induced by high-energy oxygen (hydroxide radicals) produced by selenium.

The two-step apoptotic process is illustrated in figure 4.1. In this example, selenite is functioning as the apoptotic trigger that initiates the actual execution step. Regardless of the triggering event, cellular DNA is cut into small pieces by the Ca^{+2}/ Mg^{+2}-dependent endonuclease resulting in the death of the cell.

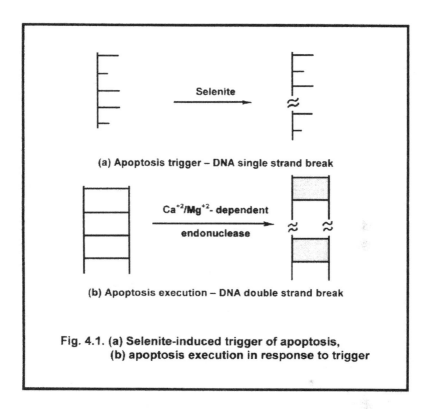

(a) Apoptosis trigger – DNA single strand break

(b) Apoptosis execution – DNA double strand break

**Fig. 4.1. (a) Selenite-induced trigger of apoptosis,
(b) apoptosis execution in response to trigger**

HT29 human colon cancer cells with mutated p53 also were found to undergo apoptosis when treated with selenite (Stewart et al. 1997). Selenite reduced cellular glutathione levels in the HT29 cells, indicating that selenite was reacting with glutathione to produce selenodiglutathione. Since HT29 cells contain mutated p53, the apoptosis observed in these cells could not have occurred via the DNA damage-recognition pathway. This finding was consistent with earlier work (Lanfear et al. 1994) and indicated that selenite must be inducing apoptosis by another mechanism.

As early as 1986, selenium dioxide, selenous acid (hydrogen selenite), and selenic acid (hydrogen selenate) were all shown to be potent inhibitors of protein kinase C isolated from human leukemia cells (Su et al. 1989). These results prompted the authors to propose that the anticarcinogenic activity of selenium might be related to its inhibition of protein kinase C.

In a study published in 1997 (Gopalakrishka, Gunimeda, and Chen 1997) it was demonstrated that selenite reacts chemically with protein kinase C, producing disulfide linkages in the catalytic domain of the enzyme that result in its inactivation. The reaction is similar to the disulfide linkages that are produced by

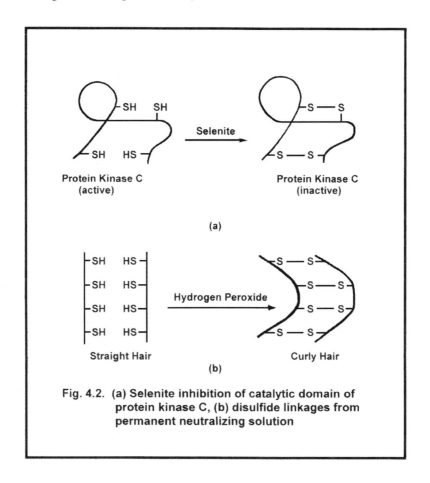

Fig. 4.2. (a) Selenite inhibition of catalytic domain of protein kinase C, (b) disulfide linkages from permanent neutralizing solution

permanent neutralizing solutions. Disulfide linkages hold the hair strands in the curled configuration dictated by the hair rollers used. Figure 4.2 illustrates the similarities between selenite inhibition of protein kinase C and the effect of neutralizing solutions on hair strands. Since the inhibition of protein kinase C is known to induce apoptosis in cancer cells (Jarvis and Grant 1997), the study revealed a plausible explanation for selenite-induced apoptosis in p53-mutated cells.

Other Anticarcinogenic Effects of Selenite

In addition to triggering apoptosis in cancer cells both by inducing DNA single-strand breaks and by inhibiting protein kinase C, selenite exerts its anticarcinogenic effects in many other ways. For example, selenite has been shown to interfere with the attachment of a carcinogen to the DNA of colon cells (Davis et al. 1999). Also, other investigators have demonstrated that selenite reduces the hyperproliferation of human colonic crypt cells in vitro caused by incubating the cells with the bile acid deoxycholic acid (Bartram et al. 1998). As we shall see in Chapter 5, selenite also potentiates the immune system by increasing phagocytic (cell-eating) activity (Aziz, Klesius, and Fransden 1984) as well as stimulating the activity of cytotoxic white blood cells (Roy et al. 1990) and natural killer cells (Talcott, Exon, and Koller 1984) that kill cancer cells by inducing apoptosis.

Se-methylselenocysteine-Induced Apoptosis in Cancer Cells

Regardless of the chemical form of dietary selenium, amounts in excess of those needed to produce regulated levels of selenoproteins (supranutritional amounts) are prepared for excretion by "methylation". Methylation produces methylselenol, dimethylselenide, and trimethylselenonium ion. At nontoxic levels of selenium intake, methylselenol is the predominant metabolite. At higher (toxic) intakes, dimethylselenide is also produced and is exhaled in the lungs imparting a garlic odor to the breath. As the level of selenium intake is increased, the amounts of dimethlyselenide and trimethylselenonium ion produced increase proportionally.

In 1990, methylated selenium metabolites were shown to have impressive anticarcinogenic activity (Ip and Ganther 1990). Later studies (Ip et al. 1991, Vadhanavikit et al. 1993) established that chemical forms of selenium with a single methyl group such as methylselenol were most likely responsible for much of the anticancer activity of selenium. Ultimately, it was established that immediate precursors of methylselenol such as methylselenocysteine, in fact, were among the most potent anticarcinogens (Ip et al. 2000a).

The shift in focus to methylated selenium compounds led to the discovery that they also trigger apoptosis in cancer cells, but in a manner distinct from selenite and selenodiglutathione. Indeed, methylselenocysteine did not produce single-strand breaks in the DNA of cancer cells to trigger apoptosis by the p53-mediated damage recognition pathway. Instead, it inhibited cell-cycle proteins (Sinha, Said, and Medina 1996), resulting in cell-cycle arrest in S-phase and apoptosis (Sinha and Medina 1997). A later study revealed that methylselenocysteine, like selenite, inhibits protein kinase C (Sinha et al. 1999). While selenite reacts directly with the catalytic domain of protein kinase C to produce disulfide bonds, methylselenocysteine's effects are likely the result of its initial metabolite methylselenol reacting with protein kinase C by one of the several mechanisms proposed by Ganther (Ganther 1999). Because methylselenocysteine does not produce DNA damage, it is intrinsically less toxic to healthy cells.

Since methylselenocysteine is present in high-selenium garlic and to a lesser degree in high-selenium yeast, it likely accounts for much of the anticancer activity in these products.

Selenomethionine,
Anticancer Activity and Apoptosis

The charcteristic of selenomethionine that sets it apart from all other dietary chemical forms of selenium is its random insertion into cellular proteins. The cell's inability to distinguish between methionine and selenomethionine results in the highest tissue levels and the lowest antitumor activity among the naturally-occurring forms of dietary selenium (Ip and Hayes 1989). That fraction of dietary selenomethionine sequestered in proteins is removed from active metabolism and is not available for producing the effective anticarcinogen methylselenol.

Evidence of the relatively poor anticancer effectiveness of selenomethionine has been presented by several investigators. In an *in vitro* study employing BALB/c MK-2 transformed mouse keratinocytes (Stewart et al 1999), sodium selenite and selenocystamine, but not selenomethionine, induced apoptosis at all dose levels investigated. Furthermore, Fischer-344 rats were used to demonstrate that dietary selenium supplements of selenite and selenate, but not selenomethionine, prevented the attachment of the carcinogen 3,2-dimethyl-4-aminobiphenyl to the DNA of colon cells (Davis et al. 1999). The implication of this study is that preventing the interaction of a carcinogen with the DNA of colon cells can prevent carcinogen-induced DNA mutations and, consequently, colon cancer.

The fact that high-selenium yeast, with most of its selenium in the form of selenomethionine, can prevent cancer in humans prompted a study designed to establish whether or not selenomethionine effectively prevented azoxymethane-induced colon cancer in F344 rats (Reddy et al. 2000). These investigators reported that dietary selenomethionine supplements had no effect on the incidence or multiplicity of azoxymethane-induced colon cancer. Consequently, it was concluded that a selenium compound other than selenomethionine must be responsible for the anticancer effectiveness of high-selenium yeast. In fact, a recent study employing high performance liquid chromatography with inductively-coupled plasma mass spectrographic detection (Ip et al. 2000b) has shown that the principal forms of selenium in high-selenium garlic and high-selenium yeast are methylselenocysteine and selenomethionine, respectively. In an effort to explain the superior anticancer activity of high-selenium garlic relative to that of high-selenium yeast, these authors suggest that removal of selenomethionine from active metabolism by insertion into tissue proteins may account for its reduced anticarcinogenic effectiveness.

In a study involving a direct comparison of the effects of methylselenocysteine with those of selenomethionine upon mouse mammary tumor cells (Sinha et al. 1999), methylselenocysteine, but not selenomethionine, inhibited the protein kinase C activity of the tumor cells. Since the inhibition of protein kinase C has been shown to be an effective method of inducing apoptosis in a variety of malignant cell types (Jarvis and Grant 1999), selenomethionine's inability to inhibit protein kinase C doubtless contributes to its lesser effectiveness as an anticancer agent.

Although selenomethionine has been reported to induce apoptosis, doses greater than those of either selenite or methylselenocysteine are required (Baines et al. 1997). Since apoptosis appears to account for much of the anticancer activity of selenium, it would seem that selenomethionine is a poor choice for cancer prevention.

Practical Aspects of Selenium-Induced Apoptosis

There is little doubt that the induction of apoptosis is critically important to the prevention and treatment of cancer. Widely used chemotherapeutic drugs such as tamoxifen, which inhibits protein kinase C (Horgan et al. 1986), and cisplatin, which activates the p53-mediated damage recognition pathway, both exert their antitumor effects by the induction of apoptosis.

A preponderance of the existing evidence indicates that much of selenium's anticarcinogenic activity is associated with its induction of apoptosis. Thus, it is extremely likely that the dietary selenium supplement that affords the greatest protection from cancer is that which most effectively induces apoptosis. Clearly, the two dietary forms that best satisfy this criterion are selenite and methylselenocysteine. As you recall, selenite induces apoptosis by both the p53-mediated damage-recognition pathway and by protein kinase C inhibition. By way of comparison, methylselenocysteine does not activate the p53-mediated damage-recognition pathway, but does inhibit protein kinase C. Selenomethionine does neither.

In Chapter 7 we shall consider other important considerations in the selection of a dietary selenium supplement such as potency, potential toxicity, and availability of the various chemical forms.

CHAPTER 5

SELENIUM-ENHANCED IMMUNITY

"Believe nothing, no matter where you read it or who has said it, not even if I have said it, unless it agrees with your own reason and your own common sense"

—Buddha

Introduction

The basis for a healthy life is an optimally-functioning immune system. That individuals with compromised immunities suffer an increased incidence of cancer is *prima facie* evidence that our cancer risk is determined, in part, by the condition of our immune system. Since immunocompetence can be impaired by aging, stress, poor nutrition, and radiation as well as various infections, it is important that we learn about and adopt those practices that enhance our immune responses. One such practice is dietary supplementation with selenite. In order to understand the considerable evidence that selenium supplements potentiate our immune defenses against cancer, we must have a rough appreciation of the nature of our immune system components that have cancer-fighting responsibility.

Our Immune Machinery

Our immune systems consist of white blood cells (leukocytes) and the proteins they produce. Leukocytes are classified according to their immune responsibilities as are immune system proteins. Table 5.1 shows the various leukocytes and the function of each. In addition to its cellular components, the immune system includes several different groups of proteins, each having a specific role in our body's response to infective agents and damaged or malignant cells. The major groups of immune system proteins and their responsibilities are detailed in table 5.2.

Table 5.1

Leukocytes and Their Immune Responsibilities

Leukocyte	Responsibilities
Phagocytes	
Neutrophils (Blood)	**Consume cells and cellular debris**
Macrophages (Tissues)	**Consume cells and cellular debris**
Natural Killer Cells (NK) Cells	**Kill cancer cells and virus-infected cells**
Basophils (Blood)	**Produce inflammation**
Mast Cells (Tissues)	**Produce inflammation**
Dendritic Cells	**Recognize infective agents and introduce them to lymphocytes**
Lymphocytes	
B-Cells	**Produce initial antibody response to Infective agents and manufacture antibodies**
T-Cells	**Produce cytokines that help B-cells make antibodies and kill virus-infected and cancer cells**
Eosinophils	**Kill parasites too big to be eaten by phagocytes**

Table 5.2

Major Immune System Protein Groups and Their Responsibilities

Protein Group	Responsibilities
Complement	Initiate inflammation, attract phagocytes, and rupture target cells
Antibodies	Identify specific infectious agents and initiate B-cell cloning to produce more antibodies
Cytokines	
Interferons	Inhibit cell proliferation and viral replication and activate phagocytes
Interleukins	Growth factor for lymphocytes, proliferate cytotoxic lymphocytes and natural killer cells, and activate phagocytes
Acute Phase Proteins	Enhance complement activation and limit damage from trauma, inflammation, malignancy, etc.

The imposing array of specialized leukocytes and immune system proteins collaborate to identify and destroy bacteria, viruses, parasites, and cancer cells, which are foreign to our bodies and pose a threat to our health.

Our Immune Defense Against Cancer

To understand selenium's role in the enhancement of our immune response to cancer cells, we need to consider only those leukocytes and immune system proteins that relate to cancer immunology. At the outset, however, we must learn how leukocytes recognize cancer cells.

All cells recognize and communicate with one another by way of proteins placed on the exterior surface of the cell by the cell's DNA. Since the DNA in the nucleus of the cell determines everything about the cell, proteins appearing on its external surface reflect the nature of the DNA in the cell's nucleus and, thus, its identity. That is, various kinds of cells are recognized by their different surface proteins. Proteins on the surface of a cell are called receptors since they "receive" (accommodate) external proteins that are precisely shaped to exactly fit into the receptor proteins. Consequently, the presence or absence of particular surface receptors allows leukocytes or antibodies to determine whether any given cell belongs in our bodies or is, in fact, a foreign invader (antigen). Once it is established that a cell is foreign, the marked invader can be destroyed in a variety of ways depending upon the leukocyte or antibody that recognizes the antigen initially.

As we discussed in Chapter 4, carcinogens, viruses, and high-energy radiation are all capable of altering (mutating) the DNA in our cells. Since cancer cells arise from the transformation of mutated cells, the DNA and, therefore, some of the receptor proteins on the surface of malignant cells differ from those on normal cells. Those receptor proteins appearing only on cancer cells are called tumor antigens and are markers used by the immune system to recognize cancer cells. Cancer cells arising from a viral infection tend to have the same tumor antigen, which is peculiar to that virus. By contrast, DNA alterations produced by carcinogens or radiation typically occur in random sites on the DNA and result in tumor antigens that differ from one cancer to another.

Cancer Cell Surveillance

Among the many components of our immune system, cytotoxic lymphocytes (CTL) and natural killer (NK) cells are primarily responsible for the recognition and destruction of virus-infected cells and cancer cells. CTL and NK cells kill on contact without relying upon help from other immune system cells. These cells exert their lethal effects by attaching to a tumor antigen on a cancer cell, cutting a hole in the cancer cell membrane, and introducing a protein-dissolving enzyme that induces apoptosis in the cancer cell. Contact with an antigen activates CTL or NK cells and results in their proliferation. Helper T-cells manufacture a lymphokine (one of the immune proteins) called interleukin-2 (IL-2) that enhances the activation of both CTL and NK cells. IL-2-activated CTL and NK cells are called tumor-infiltrating lymphocytes (TIL) and lymphokine-activated killer (LAK) cells, respectively. Other lymphokines such as IL-1 activate phagocytes, in this example macrophages, which consume the cancer cells in tissues.

Proper cancer cell surveillance depends upon adequate populations of CTL and NK cells. When our immune system is compromised by stress, etc., the numbers of these cells are decreased, and our cancer risk increases correspondingly.

If a cancer cell manages to avoid detection by CTL and NK cells, it may be recognized by a B-cell. The attachment of a B-cell to the tumor antigen of a cancer cell causes the manufacture of more B-cells capable of recognizing the cancer cell. The new B-cells manufacture antibody proteins that will bind to the same tumor antigen so that other cancer cells just like the original are also marked for destruction.

Selenium Effects on Nonspecific Immunity

Nonspecific immunity is our underlying immune system that is present in the absence of any infectious agent and is a measure of our overall ability to resist the effects of our encounters with disease-producing agents. Dietary selenium supplementation has been shown to enhance resistance to bacterial infections in many animal studies. The activity of phagocytic cells (neutrophils) in goats was significantly enhanced by selenium supplementation (Aziz, Klesius, and Fransden 1984). Neutrophil-mediated bactericidal response to *Staphylococcus aureus* in cattle also was reported (Gyang et al. 1984) to be significantly enhanced by dietary supplementation with selenium and vitamin E. In a series of studies, J. E. Spallholz, et al. reported that: selenium-supplemented mice produced greater numbers of antibodies in response to sheep red blood cell antigen than unsupplemented animals (Spallholz et al. 1973); selenium supplementation enhanced antibody production in both primary and secondary responses (Spallholz et al. 1974); antibody enhancement was greatest when the selenium supplement was given before or along with the sheep red blood cell antigen (Spallholz et al. 1975).

Effects of Selenium on Cytotoxic Lymphocytes and Natural Killer Cells

There is considerable evidence that the cancer-killing effectiveness of CTL and NK cells is enhanced by selenium supplementation. Two early studies (Talcott, Exon, and Koller 1984) and (Koller, Exon, and Talcott 1986) demonstrated that selenium supplementation enhanced cancer-cell killing by NK cells in rats. The cancer cell killing of both CTL and NK cells in mice was shown to be enhanced in selenite-supplemented mice (Petrie et al. 1989). NK cell activity was increased 70% relative to unsupplemented animals, and the response occurred more rapidly. A year later, a 22.3% increase in the CTL killing of cancer cells in selenite-supplemented mice was observed (Roy et al. 1990). The reported increase was consistent with an increase in the number of activated CTL in the lymphocyte population.

Since aging is known to impair immunity, studies have been conducted to determine selenium's impact upon the aging of the immune system. A 1995 study (Roy et al. 1995) demonstrated that the age-related reduction in CTL cancer-killing ability could be abolished in older mice by dietary selenite supplementation for a period of eight weeks. The CTL cancer-killing effectiveness of older, selenium-supplemented mice was increased by 61% relative to the unsupplemented mice, restoring the CTL cancer-killing ability to the same level as that of young adult mice. Interestingly, the increase in CTL activity occurred without a parallel increase in the lymphokine IL-2 that activates cytotoxic lymphocytes. Indeed, a separate study (L. Kiremidjian-Schumacher et al. 1992) determined that selenium supplementation increased the number of IL-2 receptors on cytotoxic lymphocytes rather than increasing IL-2 production. The study examined mice on selenium-deficient, selenium-normal, and selenium-supplemented diets to determine the effects of dietary selenium upon: the ability of stimulated lymphocytes to proliferate and produce IL-2; the ability of activated lymphocytes to produce IL-2 receptors; and the ability of macrophages (phagocytes present in tissues) to activate and produce IL-1. Mice on selenium-deficient diets showed impaired immune responses compared to mice on normal diets. The opposite was observed for selenium-supplemented animals. Selenite-supplemented mice showed an enhanced response to antigen with an increased production of CTL. Both IL-1 and IL-2 were found to be the same in mice with and without selenite supplements, but selenite-supplemented mice produced greater numbers of high-affinity IL-2 receptors. Selenite-supplemented mice also showed an enhanced ability to destroy cancer cells. The greater numbers of activated CTL and macrophage cells in selenite-supplemented animals were responsible for the observed increase in cancer-cell killing. A follow-up study conducted by the same investigators (Roy et al. 1993) demonstrated that the killing effectiveness of activated CTL cells is actually dependent upon two high-affinity receptors rather than one. As it turned out, selenite-supplementation increased the numbers of both receptors and, thus, the cell's effectiveness.

The Effects of Selenite Supplements on Human Immune Cells

In the last analysis, it is much more satisfying to know that dietary selenium supplementation can produce the same kinds of immune enhancements in humans. In 1993, Roy et al. administered 200 microgram-per-day dietary selenite supplements to research subjects whose diets were determined to be selenium-adequate prior to the start of an eight-week supplementation period (Roy et al. 1994). Other subjects with selenium-adequate diets were given placebos for comparison. After stimulation of peripheral blood lymphocytes from subjects with antigen for 48 hours, activated lymphocytes in selenite-supplemented subjects had 43.8% more high-affinity IL-2 receptors per cell compared with those from subjects receiving placebos. *In vitro* selenite supplementation of peripheral lymphocytes from selenium-adequate subjects also showed a 45.1% greater proliferation compared to unsupplemented cells.

In a companion paper resulting from the same human supplementation trial (Kiremidjian-Schumacher et al. 1994) these investigators reported their findings with respect to CTL and NK cell populations. The 200-microgram-per-day selenite supplements resulted in a 118% increase in cancer-killing ability of CTL cells and an 82.3% increase in natural killer cell activity compared to the CTL and NK cell populations from the same subjects prior to supplementation. Relative to the placebo group, the increase in the cancer-killing ability of CTL and the increase in NK cell activity were 62.8% and 108%, respectively. The number of lymphocytes required to kill a fixed number of cancer cells in the supplement group was decreased by 56.6% compared to the start of the study and 46.1% less than the placebo group. These findings clearly demonstrate that selenium supplementation above normal dietary intakes are necessary to produce enhancement of immune responses in humans.

The question of how selenium-supplementation might affect age-related impairment of immune responses in older humans also has been addressed. In 1991, a statistically significant, selenium-induced enhancement of human immune responses was demonstrated in a population of elderly institutionalized subjects (Peretz 1991). Nursing home residents above 65 years of age were given either 100-microgram-per-day selenium supplements (selenium-enriched yeast) or a placebo for six months. Prior to the start of the supplementation period, the average lymphocyte response of participating subjects to antigen stimulation was determined to be significantly below that for younger healthy adults. After four months of supplementation, the subjects receiving selenium had a 79% increase in their lymphocyte proliferation in response to antigen stimulation. Six months into the study, the lymphocyte-proliferation response of selenium-supplemented subjects had been enhanced further to 138%. This study clearly illustrates the importance of dietary selenium supplementation in the compensation for age-related decreases in human immune responses.

As we discussed in Chapter 4, chemically active forms of oxygen, produced when our cells burn the food we eat or when phagocytes kill invading cells, can contribute to cell damage. Oxygen-damaged immune system cells, of course, contribute to a reduction in immunocompetence. In 1995, E. Sun, et al., (Sun et al. 1995) demonstrated that selenite supplements prevent oxygen-induced damage to lymphocytes. Since fats (lipids) are particularly susceptible to attack by oxygen, the amount of lipid peroxide (produced from lipid/oxygen reactions) in cells is a measure of oxygen damage. These investigators used the chemically-active oxygen produced by the immune response to antigens to study the effects of selenite on the production of lipid peroxides. Selenite prevented the production of lipid peroxides in proportion to the size of selenite supplement. Thus, the preemptive reaction of oxygen with selenite prevents leukocyte damage and preserves immune competence. In a companion paper (Sun et al. 1995), the same investigators reported that selenite also prevented oxygen damage to lymphocyte immunocompetence caused by either hydrogen peroxide of the high-energy radiation from radioactive isotope cobalt-60. In their excellent review of selenium's effects on the immune system, L. Kiremidjian-Schumacher and G. Stotzky (Kiremidjian-Schumacher and Stotzky 1987) concluded that:

1. selenium deficiency is immunosuppressive
2. selenium supplementation is immunostimulatory, and
3. inorganic selenium is most effective.

CHAPTER 6

NUTRIENTS THAT INTER-ACT WITH SELENIUM

Nutrient Interactions

Just as we must be concerned with the consequences of interactions between the drugs we are taking concurrently, it is important to consider how the amounts of other substances in our cells affect the benefits that can be derived from taking supplementary nutrients such as selenium. Indeed, selenium's ability to trigger suicide in cancer cells is precisely dependent upon the interaction between selenium and other cellular components. Therefore, our choices of food and food supplements may produce either positive or negative effects upon our body's normal biochemical processes. Selenium antagonists are substances that interfere with the biological activity of selenium. Selenium synergists have the opposite effect of its antagonists in that they amplify selenium's biological effectiveness. To enjoy the greatest cancer-prevention benefit from dietary selenium supplementation, we must do what we can to avoid selenium antagonists while increasing our intake of its synergists.

The present chapter discusses how antagonists and synergists may amplify, reduce, or abolish completely the cancer-protective benefit of selenium.

Zinc

Zinc is an important dietary trace element that is essential to growth, development, reproduction, wound healing, and protein and nucleic acid biochemistry (Underwood 1977). As early as 1977, G. N. Schrauzer and his associates, using age-adjusted cancer mortalities and apparent dietary intakes of selenium, zinc, cadmium, copper, chromium, arsenic, and manganese calculated from average concentrations in major food items and per capita consumption data, investigated the relationship between cancer mortality and dietary intakes of the seven trace elements in 28 countries throughout the world (Schrauzer, White, and Schneider 1977). Among the elements studied, dietary intakes of selenium and zinc were strongly (at least 99% statistical confidence), but oppositely, associated with mortalities from cancers of the intestine, rectum, breast, prostate, lung, and leukemia. Higher dietary selenium intakes were associated with lower cancer mortalities, whereas, higher dietary zinc intakes occurred with higher cancer mortalities. These findings led them to speculate that the United States, Canada, New Zealand, Australia, and France, with the highest dietary zinc intakes among the 28 countries studied, might have zinc intakes sufficient to reduce the cancer-preventive activity of selenium.

In addition to their international study of dietary intakes and cancer, these researchers also investigated the relationship between measured blood levels of selenium, zinc, cadmium, and copper, and cancer mortalities at 19 collection sites in the United States. Their findings that high blood levels of zinc were associated with lower blood levels of selenium in the United States, led them to proposed that higher dietary zinc intakes may interfere with selenium absorption.

The dramatic impact of dietary zinc supplementation upon the cancer-preventive activity of selenium was demonstrated in the laboratory (Schrauzer, White, and Schneider 1976). Using a strain of highly inbred mice that developed spontaneous breast cancers with an incidence of

86%, these researchers compared the cancer-preventive effectiveness of a dietary selenium supplement with that of a combined selenium-zinc supplement to determine any effect zinc might have upon the cancer-preventive activity of selenium. The addition of two micrograms of selenium in the form of selenium dioxide to each liter of the mice's drinking water reduced their incidence of spontaneous breast cancers from 86% down to only 10%. When both selenium and zinc in amounts of 5 and 200 micrograms per liter, respectively, were added to the drinking water of the same strain of mouse, the spontaneous breast cancer incidence was increased to 94%. Amazingly, 200-microgram zinc supplements were sufficient to completely abolish the cancer-protective benefit of 5-microgram selenium supplements.

In light of recent research demonstrating that one of the most important ways selenium prevents cancer is by triggering cell suicide (apoptosis), zinc's interference with selenium's anticarcinogenic activity makes perfect sense. As discussed in Chapter 3, one of the essential components of any cell's suicide machinery is a calcium-magnesium dependent endonuclease that is responsible for cutting up double-stranded DNA in the execution of apoptosis. Among those engaged in research on apoptosis, it is general knowledge that zinc can be used to prevent apoptosis by blocking the activity of this endonuclease (Tanuma 1996). In fact, zinc was used to block selenite-induced DNA double-strand breaks and cell death in mouse leukemia cells (Lu et al. 1994).

Apart from its interference with apoptosis and the anticarcinogenic activity of selenium, there is evidence that zinc can enhance the proliferation of human prostate cancer. Indeed, it has been reported (Nemoto et al. 2000) that zinc enhances telomerase activity in the human prostate cancer cell line DU145 and, thereby, promotes unlimited proliferation. This finding is particularly disturbing in view of the conventional wisdom among alternative medicine enthusiasts that zinc supplements promote prostate health.

Faced with convincing evidence that supranutritional amounts of zinc are antagonistic to selenium and that the United States has one of the highest dietary zinc intakes in the world, it is enigmatic that vitamin manufacturers would choose to produce multivitamins that contain both zinc and selenium. The contents of zinc and selenium in some of these products are shown in table 6.1.

Among four of the leading brands of multivitamins examined at my local pharmacy, I discovered that the average weight ratio of zinc to selenium in these products was 545 to 1. Astonishingly, this value is much larger than the weight ratio of 40 to 1 that was reported to be sufficient to completely abolish the cancer-prevention benefit of selenium in laboratory animals (Schrauzer, White and Schneider 1976). It certainly raises some serious questions concerning the reasoning behind the inclusion of nutritional antagonists in a single multivitamin product.

Table 6.1

Zinc and Selenium Contents of Some Commercially Available Multivitamins

Component	Brand A	Brand B	Brand C	Brand D
Zinc (milligrams)	15	15	15	15
Selenium (micrograms)	87.5	21	20	0

It has been established (Schrauzer, White, and Schneider 1977) that mixed diets in the United States provide 12 to 15 milligrams of zinc per day, which agrees with their calculated value of 14 milligrams. In addition to the zinc we get from our diet, there are other less obvious sources. Carbonated drink dispensers employed in convenience stores and fast food restaurants typically have galvanized fittings connected to carbon dioxide cylinders. Such fittings as well as galvanized pipes used in plumbing applications are excellent sources of additional zinc, particularly in those geographic areas with more acidic water. Since the Recommended Dietary Allowance (RDA) published by the National Academy of Science (NAS) is 15 milligrams of zinc per day (Pennington 1989), the need for commercial dietary zinc supplements is unsupported by facts. While from a practical perspective there is no need to do anything about limiting our dietary intake of zinc, we can avoid exacerbating the problem by not taking dietary zinc supplements.

Vitamin C

Because vitamin C and selenium are both antioxidants, it is logical to suppose that combinations of vitamin C and selenium might well provide greater cancer-preventive benefit than either used individually. In attempting to determine how other potential anticarcinogens might interact with selenium, Dr. C. Ip administered dietary supplements of selenium, vitamin C, as well as a selenium-vitamin C combination to rats (Ip 1987). Other rats were given no dietary supplement for comparison. All rats were also given dimethlybenzanthracene (DMBA) to induce breast cancers. Rats given 4 micrograms of selenium in each gram of food had a 40% breast cancer incidence, which was 36% lower than that for the unsupplemented control rats. Rats given 5-milligram vitamin C supplements in each gram of food suffered an 80% incidence of breast cancer, which was statistically indistinguishable from the unsupplemented rats. Surprisingly, rats supplemented with a combination of the selenium and vitamin C given in the same doses used in the individual supplements experienced a 68% incidence of breast cancer, which was higher than that of rats receiving only selenium. The interference of vitamin C with the cancer-preventive effectiveness of selenium was the precise opposite of the result expected.

The explanation for the interference of vitamin C with the cancer-preventive effectiveness of selenium is that selenite and vitamin C react to produce elemental selenium. The reaction is easy to demonstrate. Introducing a couple of powdered, or better still, dissolved sodium selenite tablets into a glass of water with a gram or so of dissolved vitamin C produces a red cloud of elemental selenium. The elemental selenium is not harmful, but it does not dissolve in water and is not metabolized. Thus, selenium from sodium selenite and vitamin C taken together may remain in the gastrointestinal tract and confer no cancer-preventive benefit.

Although no studies have been conducted on the subject, it is likely that moderate vitamin C supplements (i.e.100 to 500 milligrams) taken several hours apart from a selenite supplement would have little effect on the selenite.

Vitamin A

Using the same experimental design as that employed for the vitamin C study, Dr. Ip investigated the cancer-prevention effectiveness of supplements containing selenium alone, vitamin A alone, and a combination of selenium and vitamin A (Ip 1987). As in the vitamin C study, the dose of selenium used in supplements was 4 micrograms per gram of food. The dose of vitamin A used was 250 micrograms per gram of food. As in the vitamin C study, DMBA was given to all rats to produce breast cancer. The breast cancer incidences of rats receiving the selenium, vitamin A, and combined selenium-vitamin A supplements were reduced relative to the control rats by 36.5%, 43.3% and 73.4%, respectively. Although the combined selenium—vitamin A supplement was extremely effective in preventing breast cancers, the combination was poorly tolerated by the rats, resulting in decreased food consumption and weight loss.

In 1983, Dr. W. C. Willett, et al. published the results of their epidemiological study, which demonstrated that vitamin A improved the cancer prevention benefit of selenium in humans (Willett et al 1983). A total of 10,940 research subjects varying from 30-69 years of age were enrolled in the study. Blood samples were taken and participating research subjects were determined to be cancer free by physical examination at the beginning of the study. Subjects were monitored for five years, during which time 111 subjects developed new cancers. For each subject that developed cancer, two subjects matched as closely as possible in age, sex, race, smoking history, month of blood collection, initial blood pressure, antihypertensive medication, etc. were selected for comparison. Serum levels of selenium, vitamin A, and vitamin E were measured for the 111 subjects with cancer and the 222 cancer-free cohorts. Subjects having serum selenium levels in the lowest third of those measured had twice the cancer risk of the subjects in the highest third. Subjects with serum levels of both selenium and vitamin A in the lowest third of those measured had 3.9 times the cancer risk of the subjects in the highest third of selenium and vitamin A levels. Thus, higher selenium intakes alone reduced cancer risk by 50%, while higher intakes of both selenium and vitamin A produced a 75% risk reduction.

Vitamin E

In the same study (Willett et al. 1983) the association of combined blood levels of selenium and vitamin E upon the risk of cancer was considered. Individuals with serum levels of both selenium and vitamin E in the lowest third of all subjects had a cancer risk 2.4 times greater than subjects with serum levels in the highest third. Therefore, higher serum levels of selenium and vitamin E reduced subject's cancer risk by 68% compared to the 50% risk reduction occurring with higher serum selenium levels alone. Interestingly, subjects with serum levels in the highest third of measured selenium, vitamin A, and vitamin E had a cancer risk reduction of 84% relative to subjects with levels in the lowest third of these nutrients.

P. M. Horvath and C. Ip investigated the cancer-preventive effectiveness of dietary supplements of selenium, vitamin E, and a selenium-vitamin E combination (Horvath and Ip 1983). Rats were divided into four groups, with one group receiving no supplement and serving as the control. The other three groups were given 2.5 micrograms of selenium per gram of food, 1,000 micrograms of vitamin E per gram of food, and a combination of selenium and vitamin E administered in the same doses as the separate supplements. All groups received dimethylbenzanthracene to induce breast cancers. Cancer incidence in rats on the selenium-supplemented diet was 17% lower than that of the control group, but the reduction in cancer incidence was not large enough to be statistically significant (i.e. 95% confidence). No reduction of cancer incidence occurred in the group fed the vitamin E-supplemented diet. However, those rats given the diet supplemented with both selenium and vitamin E experienced a 33% reduction in cancer incidence. Thus, even though vitamin E alone had no effect upon the incidence of breast cancer, it synergistically increased the cancer-preventive effectiveness of the selenium supplement.

Vitamin E was also observed to enhance the cancer-preventive effectiveness of selenium in an epidemiological study conducted in eastern Finland (Salonen et al. 1985). Blood samples were taken from some 12,000 cancer-free research subjects aged 30-64 years. In the subsequent four years of follow-up, 51 subjects died of cancer. For each of the 51 subjects who died of cancer, a control subject, matched in age, sex, and smoking frequency, was selected.

Subjects with serum selenium levels in the lowest third of measured values had 5.8 times the risk of fatal cancer as those with serum selenium levels among the highest third. Subjects having serum levels of both selenium and vitamin E in the lowest third of measured values had a fatal cancer risk 11.4 times that of subjects with both selenium and vitamin E levels in the highest third.

The evidence presented in this chapter suggests that dietary supplementation with zinc or vitamin C could potentially reduce or abolish completely the cancer-prevention effectiveness of a selenium supplement. Since the typical diet in the United States provides the RDA for zinc and since there is no evidence of wide spread zinc deficiency, dietary zinc supplementation for a healthy American doesn't really make much sense.

In the case of vitamin C, the selenium antagonism appears to be related to the conversion of selenite to elemental selenium when vitamin C comes in direct contact with selenite (i.e. when they are taken together). Presumably, this would not be a problem if selenium were taken as selenomethionine. However, since selenomethionine is a much less effective anticarcinogen than selenite, the substitution of selenomethionine for selenite as a dietary supplement doesn't seem to be a sensible option. Perhaps a better approach might be to take a modest (100-200 milligrams) vitamin C supplement at breakfast and a selenium supplement with dinner in the evening. Alternatively, one could depend upon getting his RDA of vitamin C solely from his or her food. Obviously, it would be better to have data that could shed some light on the possibility of taking selenite and vitamin C and different times of the day without sacrificing the cancer prevention effectiveness of selenite.

The existing data consistently show that both vitamin A and vitamin E contribute to the cancer-preventive effectiveness of selenium. Since vitamin E occurs in foods in relatively small amounts that are typically high in fat (butter, eggs, milk, etc.) and since most of us are trying to reduce our intake of fats, it is easier to take a dietary supplement to get an sufficiently large amount of this vitamin. In my opinion, it is wiser to take vitamin E in an individual supplement rather than in a multivitamin. Too often, multivitamins include selenium antagonists that reduce or abolish selenium's cancer-preventive effectiveness.

Vitamin A is a different matter. One should be cautious about taking vitamin A supplements. A diet including yellow and orange fruits and vegetables typically supplies ample amounts of β-carotene (provitamin A). Your body converts β-carotene into the vitamin A you need, and, unlike vitamin A, is not toxic when taken in too great an amount. Indeed, since excess vitamin A has been shown to produce birth defects (Snyder 1998), pregnant women should only take vitamin A supplements when advised to do so by their physicians.

CHAPTER 7

INFORMED SELENIUM SUPPLEMENTATION

> *"Remember, then, that it [science] is the guide of action; that the truth which it arrives at is not that which we can ideally contemplate without error, but that which we may act upon without fear..."*
>
> —William Kingdon Clifford

Introduction

Our use of vitamin and mineral supplements in the United States is based, for the most part, on no data at all. In virtually all instances, we have no clue about the amount of any given vitamin or mineral we are actually getting from our food and drink. In the face of this ignorance, we proceed to supplement our diet with a variety of commercial products. Our favorite dietary insurance product is the multivitamin (the more multiple the better) that we believe covers all possible deficiencies without having to think about the matter.

Two important questions arising from such a haphazard practice are:

1. Are we doing ourselves any real harm?
2. Are we improving our health materially?

In my opinion, the answer to the first question is probably not in most instances. The most prevalent harm is likely financial. Although the ingestion of too much of the fat-soluble vitamins such as A, D, E, and K produces toxicity, very few people manage to supplement their diets with toxic amounts. With respect to the second question, I think that there is a good chance that our health is improved by many dietary supplements. While one can cite a few counterexamples, certainly there are numerous scientifically-valid studies indicating that higher blood levels of vitamins A, C, and E afford some measure of protection from some serious chronic diseases (Salonen et al. 1985).

Hopefully, the information presented in previous chapters is sufficiently compelling that you are contemplating supplementing your own diet with selenium to reduce your risk of cancer. If so, you should know that selenium, like the fat-soluble vitamins, is toxic when taken in inappropriately-large amounts. To insure that your dietary supplement is both safe and effective for the intended purpose, there are several relevant facts to consider. You should know that the several chemical forms of dietary selenium differ significantly in their anticancer potency so that the supplementary amounts required for effective protection differ correspondingly. For safety reasons, it is important to know the effects and symptoms of selenium toxicity (selenosis) and the amounts of each of the dietary chemical forms that produce selenosis symptoms in humans. With the array of commercial products available, a knowledge of the contents of each product is also important. The present chapter is intended to provide all the information you would need to make an informed choice of a dietary selenium supplement.

Determining How Much Selenium You Need

In 1989, the Food and Nutrition Board of the United States National Academy of Sciences published its first Recommended Dietary Allowance (RDA) for selenium (Levander 1991). The selenium RDA was based upon the amount of dietary selenium needed to make the essential selenoproteins and was calculated to be 70 micrograms per day for men and 55 micrograms per day for women. The RDA represents the **minimum** amount needed to avoid deficiency disease. As you may recall from Chapter 3, the amount of dietary selenium greater than that needed to manufacture the metabolically-regulated selenoproteins is referred to as a supranutritional dose and results in the conversion of excess selenium into forms suitable for excretion. You may also recall that one of the excretory forms methylselenol is a good anticarcinogen that is not produced in significant amounts unless supranutritional doses are taken. Thus, optimal cancer prevention with selenium supplements depends upon taking more than the RDA but less than the amount that produces toxicity.

To avoid inadvertently producing selenosis from dietary supplementation, we must know the minimum daily dose that produces symptoms of toxicity and the approximate amount of selenium we are already getting from our food and drink. To take the greatest supranutritional amount of selenium, we simply supplement our normal dietary intake with enough selenium to increase our total intake to just below that required to produce symptoms of toxicity. Reliable estimates of normal dietary intakes can be made from selenium data available in the United States so that we can be confident that we are safely and effectively reducing our risk of several kinds of cancer.

Estimating Your Daily Dietary Selenium Intake

Beginning with the decade of the '70s, researchers began publishing daily dietary intakes of selenium and other trace elements in countries throughout the world. Dietary intakes are estimated from the selenium contents of typical dishes in each country, from selenium levels measured in human blood and urine, and from selenium analyses of food samples taken from food actually consumed by human research subjects. Table

7.1 details some daily dietary selenium intakes at locations in the United States and Canada that have been published in the peer-review scientific and medical literature. Careful scrutiny of the research papers from which the data in table 7.1 are derived reveals some important facts. First, the difference between the selenium intakes for women from Canada and Ontario (Gibson and Scythes 1984) illustrates the importance of the method used for estimating dietary selenium intake. The value of 168 micrograms of selenium per day was calculated using published selenium levels in foods of a typical woman's diet in Canada. The value of 77 micrograms per day was determined by selenium analysis of the food actually consumed by the research subjects participating in their study. These investigators found that the actual selenium intake of research subjects was always significantly lower (statistically) than that calculated from published selenium values for the food consumed. Second, it is useful to notice that the rather substantial differences in selenium intake between geographic locations roughly correspond to the adequate, marginal, and deficient selenium regions depicted in figure 2.2 of Chapter 2. Thus, individuals living in the Central and Northern Rocky Mountain states as well as the North Central Plains states (i.e. Wyoming, Nebraska, North and South Dakota) could expect their daily dietary selenium intakes to be in

Table 7.1

Daily Dietary Selenium Intakes in the United States and Canada

Location	Daily Dietary Selenium (micrograms)	Data Source
United States	134	(Watkinson 1974)
United States	168	(Schrauzer, White, and Schneider 1977)
United States	170	(Levander 1982)
United States	108	(Pennington et al. 1974)
Oregon	70-85	(Butler and Whanger 1987)
Maryland	81	(Levander and Morris 1984)
South Dakota	216	(Olsen and Palmer 1978)
Texas	60	(Drake and Hain 1994)
Canada	77-168	(Gibson and Scythes 1984)
Wyoming	77	(Valentine et al. 1987)

the 200-microgram range. Similarly, those living on the East or West coasts or the Midwestern states might reasonably estimate their dietary selenium intakes to be in the 60- to 100-microgram-per-day range. To be sure, such values are estimates. However, they are based upon data that are self-consistent and are far better than no data at all. A few locations with small populations in high-selenium regions have selenium intakes above

200 micrograms per day. Red Butte and Jade Hills of Wyoming, Grants, New Mexico (Valentine et al. 1987), and several small communities near Rapid City, South Dakota (Robinson 1982) are representative of such high-selenium areas. Doubtless, there are others.

Anticancer Potency of the Chemical Forms of Dietary Selenium

Among the most common forms of dietary selenium, selenite and methylselenocysteine appear to have very comparable anticancer potencies. Although *in vitro* studies (Lu et al. 1996, Sinha, Said, and Medina 1996) have shown selenite to be 10 to 40 times more effective than methylselenocysteine in cancer cell inhibition, the two compounds appear to have about the same anticancer potency *in vivo* (Ip, Lisk, and Stoewsand 1992). The disparity between the *in vivo* and *in vitro* anticancer effectiveness appears to be related to the availability of the enzyme β-lyase. The conversion of methylselenocysteine into the potent anticarcinogen methylselenol requires β-lyase, which is more available in the intact organism than in cell cultures.

Ironically, the most abundant naturally-occurring chemical form of dietary selenium selenomethionine is the least potent in the prevention of cancer. In 1980, selenomethionine provided the least protection from live Ehrlich ascites tumor cell injections into the peritoneum of rats among equal doses of five chemical forms of selenium examined (Greeder and Milner 1980). Recent studies have shown that selenomethionine does not induce apoptosis in cancer cells by the DNA damage pathway (Stewart et al. 1999) or by inhibition of protein kinase C (Sinha et al. 1999). Furthermore, dietary supplementation with 2.0 parts per million selenium as selenite or selenate, but not selenomethionine, prevented the attachment of the carcinogen 3,2'-dimethyl-4-aminobiphenyl to the DNA of colonic crypt epithelial cells (Davis et al. 1999). In addition, dietary selenomethionine supplements at levels of 10 and 15 parts per million were shown to have no effect upon either the incidence or multiplicity of azoxymethane-induced colon cancers in rats (Reddy et al. 2000). It is very likely that the random incorporation of selenomethionine into cellular proteins accounts for its lack of efficacy as an anticarcinogen.

In light of the differences in anticancer potency of the several chemical forms of dietary selenium, we can best reduce our cancer risk by choosing foods or food supplements that contain smaller amounts of selenomethionine and larger amounts of selenite or methylselenocysteine.

About Selenium Toxicity

The current research pertaining to the anticancer effects of selenium is directed toward identifying the chemical forms that are most toxic to cancer cells while having the least toxicity to normal healthy cells. The expression of certain oncogenes (e.g. c-myc, E1A and ras) that produce unregulated proliferation in abnormal cells dramatically increases their susceptibility to apoptosis (Lowe 1996). Such cells are said to be primed and undergo apoptosis under conditions that only arrest cell growth in normal cells.

This is wonderful news because many selenium compounds are apoptotic agents. Consequently, selenite and methylselenocysteine, which trigger apoptosis most effectively, will always be more toxic to premalignant and malignant cells that to normal cells. We can make good use of the fact that it is easier to induce apoptosis in cancer cells than in normal cells.

In sufficiently large doses, all selenium compounds are toxic to normal cells. Generally speaking, those chemical forms that produce large amounts of hydrogen selenide (e.g. selenite) are more toxic than those that do not (methylselenocysteine, selenomethionine, etc.). Instances of human selenium toxicity (selenosis) are uncommon, having occurred in

South Dakota in the 1940s (Lemly and Merryman 1941) and during a severe drought in Enshi County, China, in the 1960s (Yang et al. 1983).

Selenium typically affects hair, skin, nails, gastrointestinal tract, and the nervous system (Chen and Clark 1986, Olsen 1986). Early signs of selenosis include: nausea, loss of hair, nail abnormalities, and breath with a garlic odor. Initial nail changes (particularly thumbnails) include white spots and longitudinal ridges, brittleness, and eventually, nail loss. New nails are thick, brittle, and rough. Individuals with selenosis often develop rashes and, with prolonged intakes of very large doses of selenium, may experience tingling or numbness in their extremities, impaired motor control, or some degree of paralysis.

Among the chemical forms of selenium used most commonly in selenium supplementation trials, selenite has generated the greatest concern about toxicity. Selenite-induced apoptosis in some cancer cells is associated with single strand breaks in DNA (Lu et al. 1994) and the generation of superoxide anion (Stewart et al. 1997). Of course, these are exactly the types of effects that contribute to the potent cancer-prevention effectiveness of selenite. The toxicity concerns are that high dose levels of selenite might be capable of producing similar lethal effects in normal cells.

There are many *in vitro* human cell culture studies demonstrating that selenite levels sufficient to induce death in cancer cells have little or no effects on normal, healthy cells. As early as 1984, evidence was presented to show that selenite levels, which induced the death of 55% of MCF-7 human breast cancer cells in 72 hours, had no effect on MRC-5 normal diploid human cells over the same period of time (Watrach et al. 1984). In a later study (Pung, Mei, and Yu 1987) human lung cancer cells incubated with a modest dose of sodium selenite exhibited a reduction in mitotic index, decrease in growth rate, and a partial inhibition of cell cycle progression, while an identical dose of sodium selenite produced no effects on human embryonic lung diploid cells. The same investigators (Pung, Mei, and Yu 1987) reported that human liver cancer cells, treated with doses of sodium selenite that were non-toxic to normal embryonic human liver cells, reduced the growth rate and inhibited the progression of the cell cycle in human liver cancer cells. Yet another study (Zhu et al. 1996), employing A172 and T98G human brain cancer cell lines, demonstrated that sodium selenite doses sufficient to inhibit proliferation and induce apoptosis in both brain cancer cell lines had little effect upon human fibroblast NT14 cells.

Although *in vitro* studies are useful in predicting the likelihood of a particular supplement being safe and effective, ultimately, we must rely only on actual human intervention trials. The result of a five-year sodium selenite-supplementation trial in Qidong county of Jiang-su province, China, was published in 1991 (Yu et al. 1991). The trial was intended to test the effect of dietary selenium supplementation upon the incidence of primary liver cancer. Sodium selenite in at a level of 15 parts per million was added to the table salt of 20,847 residents of a single township. Four neighboring townships, having a collective population of 109,624 and receiving no selenium, served as the control group. By the fifth year of the study, the age-adjusted incidence of primary liver cancer in subjects receiving sodium selenite supplements was reduced by 34% compared to the 12-year average incidence experienced by the same township before the beginning of the study. The average age-adjusted incidence of primary liver cancer over the five-year period of the study in the selenium-supplemented township also was reduced by 43% relative to that of the control group over the same five-year time period. These impressive results were achieved with no reports of selenium toxicity in the township receiving selenite supplements.

Literally millions of people in ten low-selenium provinces of China have been supplemented with sodium selenite continuously for periods varying from five to ten years without reports of selenosis or chronic health effects (Chen and Clark 1986). Certainly, the existing data suggest that dietary selenium supplementation with sodium selenite can be effective in reducing the incidence of cancer at doses that produce no negative health effects in humans.

The Maximum Safe Daily Selenium Intake

Safe daily intakes of selenium are estimated by measuring selenium intakes of people both with and without symptoms of selenosis and by studies with selenium supplementation (Chen and Clark 1986). Estimates of safe daily intakes have been determined from studies of individuals living in geographic regions with lengthy exposures to unusually high levels of naturally occurring selenium. Beginning in 1985, G. Yang, et al., studied selenium intake and its effects upon the health of inhabitants of low-, medium-, and high-selenium regions of China (Yang et al. 1989a, Yang et al. 1989b). They concluded that daily selenium intakes of 750 to 850 micrograms were marginally safe, and intakes of 400 micrograms were completely safe. M. L. Longnecker, et al., studied the selenium intake and health of people residing in high-selenium areas of eastern Wyoming and western South Dakota (Longnecker et al. 1991). After conducting physical examinations, compiling reported symptoms, and conducting numerous laboratory measurements of biochemical parameters, these investigators reported no evidence of selenium toxicity below intakes of 724 micrograms of selenium per day. Valentine et al. compared physical symptoms reported by subjects residing in geographic regions of the United States with high and normal levels of selenium in their drinking water (Valentine et al. 1987). In this instance, the chemical form of selenium ingested would have been predominantly selenite or selenate rather than the organic forms found in foods. After measuring selenium levels in hair, blood, urine, and drinking water of participating subjects to determine daily selenium intakes, the investigators reported no evidence of selenium toxicity up to daily intakes of 988 micrograms per day. In his paper reviewing the literature on selenium toxicity, O. E. Olsen suggested a maximum safe multiple oral selenium dose of five micrograms per kilogram of body weight, which corresponds to a daily dose of 350 micrograms for a 150-lb. adult (Olsen 1986). Based upon instances of chronic selenosis and experience with selenium supplementation trials, daily dose ranges of 450-900 micrograms and 750-4,990 micrograms of selenium as sodium selenite and organic selenium, respectively, were proposed (Chen and Clark 1986) for use in Phase 1 clinical trials to test selenium's cancer-prevention efficacy. The lower dose range for sodium selenite takes into consideration its greater toxicity. The United States Environmental Protection Agency has established a NOAEL (**NO A**dverse **E**ffects **L**evel) and a LOAEL (**LO**west **A**dverse **E**ffects **L**evel) for selenium intake of 0.015 and 0.023 milligram per kilogram of body weight per day, respectively (United States Environmental Protection Agency 1989). For comparison purposes, these values correspond to 853 and 1,261 micrograms per day. Estimated safe daily intakes of selenium are summarized in table 7.2. Most of the estimates of safe daily selenium intakes fall between 400 and 900 micrograms. The lower values normally include extra margins of safety to take into account variations among individuals or locations. With the exception of those very few people living in isolated, high-selenium regions of the Rocky Mountain or Northern Plains states, the maximum daily intake from food and drink would be near 200 micrograms per day. Depending upon how conservative we are in our estimates of safe daily intakes, safe selenium supplements could range from 200 to 500 micrograms per day. Obviously, those living in selenium deficient regions would opt for larger supplements than those residing in the higher selenium regions. The really exciting news is that the dramatic decreases in the incidences of lung, colorectal, and lung cancers demonstrated by Dr. Clark's double-blind, placebo-controlled clinical trial (Clark et al. 1996) were achieved with the smallest suggested level of selenium supplementation (200 micrograms per day).

Table 7.2

Estimated Maximum Safe Daily Dietary Intakes of Selenium

Safe Intake (micrograms per day)		Data Source
750-850	(marginally safe)	(Yang et al. 1989b)
400	(completely safe)	(Yang et al. 1989b)
724		(Longnecker et al. 1991)
988		(Valentine et al. 1987)
350		(Olsen 1986)
450-900	(selenite)	(Chen and Clark 1986)
750-4,990	(organic)	(Chen and Clark 1986)
853	(NOAEL)	(United States Environmental Protection Agency 1989)

Who Should Consider Dietary Selenium Supplementation?

If the advantage of dietary selenium supplementation in the United States is the reduction of cancer risk, it is clear that the real concern occurs later in life. If we are to believe data from the National Cancer Institute,

90% of all cancers occur in the 55-and-up age group. While childhood cancers are terrible tragedies, they occur less frequently, and we seldom give them conscious thought. Similarly, cancers among young adults in the child-bearing-and-rearing age group are also less common.

Information pertaining to children, pregnant women, and younger adults with greater-than-average selenium intakes is very limited. Furthermore, selenium supplementation among children, for the most part, has been confined to those geographic regions (e.g. some parts of China) where environmental levels of selenium are so low that its deficiency resulted in Keshan disease (an endemic cardiomyopathy).

In the absence of valid studies providing evidence of deficiency disease, dietary selenium supplementation in the United States among persons younger than 45 years old really makes little sense.

Commercially Available Selenium Supplements

Anyone who has ventured into a retail store that sells vitamin, mineral, and herbal supplements must be impressed by the intimidating variety of choices. If you are buying a selenium supplement, you will find selenium in multivitamins, in antioxidant formula products, with vitamin E, as selenium yeast (high-selenium yeast), as yeast-free selenium, and as sodium selenite. Each of these categories of product will include an array of similar supplements with varying amounts of selenium or with a different combination of ingredients. Faced with such a confusing assortment of products, how can one choose, with some degree of confidence, the supplement that will reduce his or her cancer risk most effectively? The following sections of this chapter are intended to provide the required information. For simplicity, I shall discuss the selection procedure as a series of five steps.

Step 1: Knowing the Chemical Form of Selenium You Want

Maybe appropriately, identifying the particular known chemical form of selenium that is most effective in preventing cancer is the easiest step in the process. The three most common chemical forms of dietary selenium are sodium selenite, methylselenocysteine, and selenomethionine. The body of existing evidence supports the conclusion that both selenite and methylselenocysteine are more effective in cancer prevention than selenomethionine. If one could choose between selenite and methylselenocysteine, the latter would be preferable because it is less toxic to healthy cells, yet it is better than, or equal to, selenite in cancer prevention. So assuming that all are commercially available, the order of preference would be:

1. methylselenocysteine
2. sodium selenite
3. selenomethionine.

Step 2: Knowing the Chemical Compositions of Commercially-Available Supplements

Organic forms of selenium such as selenomethionine or methylselenocysteine are usually obtained from either yeast or garlic that is grown in a medium containing some inorganic form of selenium such as selenium dioxide, sodium selenite, or sodium selenate. Oganisms convert inorganic selenium into the organic forms they need. Although both yeast and garlic manufacture several forms of organic selenium, one form typically predominates over the others. The most recent and accurate chemical analysis of high-selenium yeast and high-selenium garlic was conducted using a very sensitive analytical technique called high-performance liquid chromatography with inductively-coupled plasma mass spectrometry or with electrospray mass spectrometry (Ip et al. 2000). These researchers reported that 73% of the selenium in high-selenium garlic is present as γ-glutamyl-Se-methylselenocysteine and 85% of the selenium in high-selenium yeast is selenomethionine. In addition to the analytical work, these investigators conducted dietary supplementation studies involving rats given various doses of either high-selenium yeast or high-selenium garlic. Tissue selenium levels were always higher in rats given high-selenium yeast supplements. However, when the rats were treated with a carcinogen to produce breast cancers, those receiving high-selenium garlic had lower incidences of both premalignant lesions and breast cancers. The poorer cancer protection afforded by the high-selenium yeast was attributed to the random insertion of selenomethionine into tissue proteins. Although selenomethionine comprises the greatest fraction of the selenium in high-selenium yeast, methylselenocysteine, selenocystine, and selenoethionine collectively account for approximately 20% of the supplement (Bird et al. 1997).

Because of its large methylselenocysteine content, high-selenium garlic is far superior to high-selenium yeast as a cancer-prevention supplement. Regrettably, there are no high-selenium garlic dietary supplements commercially available at the time of this writing. In fact, the overwhelming majority of all commercial selenium supplements presently available contain high-selenium yeast. The large selenomethionine content of high-selenium yeast makes it one of the poorer dietary selenium supplements from the standpoint of cancer prevention.

Yeast-free supplements are manufactured and marketed for individuals who are allergic to yeast. Unfortunately, most of these supplements contain 100% selenomethionine and, therefore, would be a very poor choice for reducing the risk of cancer. The prevailing wisdom that anything organic is good coupled with ignorance of the facts about selenium allows such products to be successful enough to remain on the market. Of course, those selling such supplements would argue that they are intended to provide the RDA for selenium rather than for preventing cancer. A quick glance at table 7.1 is sufficient to invalidate that argument, since dietary selenium intakes in the United States already provide the RDA of selenium. The sole justifiable reason for taking supplementary selenium is to provide sufficient amounts to prevent cancer effectively.

At present, the commercially-available selenium supplement containing all of its selenium in a form that effectively prevents cancer is sodium selenite. In spite of its excellent cancer-prevention effectiveness, it is among the most difficult to find in stores. When taken in non-toxic amounts, selenite should afford the greatest cancer protection benefit among the commercial supplements currently available.

Step 3: Eliminating Products That Have Little or None of the Chemical Form You Want

Multivitamins and antioxidant formula products contain selenium, but they typically contain such small amounts of selenium that they could not be effective in cancer prevention. The prophylactic benefit from selenium supplements increases with dosage so that the low doses provided by these products would be expected to confer little or no measurable protection. To make matters worse, even the small amounts of selenium present in such supplements are usually in the form of selenomethionine. Other valid reasons for eliminating these products from consideration are discussed in Step 4.

Step 4: Eliminating Products with Selenium Antagonists

In Chapter 4 we considered the peer-reviewed scientific evidence that excessive intakes of zinc can abolish the cancer preventive effectiveness of selenium. Selenium and zinc have opposite effects upon apoptosis in pre-malignant and malignant cells. While selenium induces apoptosis by several different mechanisms, higher zinc levels inhibit the endonuclease enzyme essential for the death of these cells. There is little doubt that zinc is a powerful selenium antagonist.

Since people in the United States already get the RDA for zinc in their diets, zinc supplementation is non-productive at best and, at worst, may be counterproductive to reducing one's cancer risk. Virtually all antioxidant formulas and multivitamins contain substantial amounts of zinc, and, consequently, can be eliminated as possible choices for selenium supplementation regardless of the chemical form of selenium used in these supplements.

Step 5: Select from Remaining Products Based Upon Their Effectiveness

Considering both cancer-preventive effectiveness and toxicity, high-selenium garlic or a selenium supplement consisting of 100% methylselenocysteine would be the best choices. Unfortunately, neither of these products is commercially available and both must be eliminated as possibilities. Among commercial products that are available, multivitamins, antioxidant formulas, and yeast-free selenium supplements have been eliminated because they contain too little selenium, or an ineffective form of selenium, or they contain selenium antagonists.

Only two choices remain for consideration as possible selenium supplements: sodium selenite and high-selenium yeast. Based upon the most recent analytical information we can estimate that high-selenium yeast is approximately 80% selenomethionine and 20% of assorted selenoamino acids including methylselenocysteine. Dr. Clark's ten-year, double-blind clinical trial (Clark et al. 1996) established that high-selenium yeast can reduce cancer risk in humans. These results are surprisingly good considering that the greatest fraction of the selenium in high selenium yeast is selenomethionine. Indeed, the inability of selenomethionine to prevent azoxymethane-induced colon cancers at dietary levels as high as 15 parts per million (Reddy et al. 2000) led to the conclusion that some selenium compound other than selenomethionine was responsible for the cancer prevention effectiveness of high-selenium yeast.

The Take-Home Message Concerning Dietary Selenium Supplementation

There is little remaining ambiguity concerning the safety and cancer-preventive effectiveness of dietary selenium supplementation. Apart from considerations about the most effective chemical form, it is important to understand that the amount of dietary selenium is critical to the successful reduction of your cancer risk. Unless you are in that minute fraction of the population living in an area with very high levels of environmental selenium, you cannot rely on your diet, no matter how healthy it is, to provide you with sufficient selenium to reduce your cancer risk below that of the general population. In order for selenium to have any material impact on your cancer risk in the later years of your life, you must opt for some dietary supplement. As with any practice that impacts your health, you should consult your physician to establish that selenium supplements are appropriate for you before you start your new supplementation regimen.

Purchasing the selenium supplement you want is easy. Be sure to buy a supplement that contains only selenium. If you prefer high-selenium yeast, you can find this selenium supplement in virtually any store that sells nutritional supplements. Most people buying nutritional products think that organic forms of everything are better, so such products are easy to sell. If there is any mention of yeast on the label, e.g. selenized yeast, selenium in yeast, selenium-enriched yeast, or high-selenium yeast, they are all essentially the same product.

If, on the other hand, you prefer sodium selenite, finding a source will be more difficult. You may be able to get your nutritional supplement store to order it for you. Chain stores many times will not do that because they stock only their own brands of vitamins and minerals and their in-house brand does not include sodium selenite. If your normal source of vitamins and minerals doesn't carry and cannot order sodium selenite, your next best option is the internet. Simply type in "sodium selenite" in any internet search engine and you can immediately find several sources.

Selenium supplements vary from 50 to 200 micrograms per tablet or capsule. You can choose the size that is most convenient to use based upon the daily supplement you want.

In the event that you and your physician agree that selenium supplementation is appropriate for you, be sure to do it every day. Since it is the metabolic products of the dietary forms of selenium that are responsible for the cancer-preventive properties of selenium rather than the dietary forms themselves, it is important to generate a continuous level of these metabolites.

Afterword

Understanding the many ways in which dietary selenium supplementation can contribute to the reduction of cancer risk in humans, it is both tempting and incorrect to conclude or assume that daily, supranutritional intakes of selenium will compensate for lifestyle choices that increase cancer risk. Smoking or other uses of tobacco, excessive alcohol consumption, exposing our bodies unnecessarily to UV or X-ray radiation, and consistent consumption of high-fat foods or daily high-calorie diets all correlate significantly with increased cancer incidence in humans. These practices are associated with exposure to larger amounts of carcinogens or increased cellular damage from oxygen and, consequently, a proportionally greater risk of cancer.

Ultimately, the effective minimization of cancer risk beyond middle age depends upon both reducing our exposure to carcinogens and increasing our intake of anticarcinogens. Common sense tells us that a partial commitment to preventive measures will produce partially successful results. Having said that, conscientiously choosing to forgo an easy, inexpensive, and potentially life-extending practice such as dietary supplementation with the proven anticarcinogen selenium seems irrational.

No matter how conscientiously and completely we adhere to a low-cancer-risk lifestyle, we cannot be assured of avoiding cancer in our lifetimes. What we can do with certainty is dramatically reduce the likelihood that we will be stricken by the disease.

Over time, more effective cancer therapies will be developed and implemented. You can be sure, however, they will be more costly, in every regard, than dietary selenium supplementation.

Glossary

Aflatoxin B$_1$ A toxin produced by the fungus *Aspergillis Flavus,* which grows on corn, wheat, and peanuts in hot, damp climates.

Antagonist A substance that interferes with the normal biological activity of something else.

Antibody A protein that identifies a specific infectious agent and marks it for destruction.

Anticarciongen A substance that prevents and/or inhibits cancer.

Antigen An infective agent.

Apoptosis A genetically controlled cell suicide.

Atom The smallest particle comprising any element.

Basal cell carcinoma The least aggressive skin cancer.

Basophil A white blood cell that produces inflammation.

B-cell Produces initial antibody response to infective agent and manufactures antibodies.

Benzo(a)pyrene A carcinogen in smoke.

Butylated hydroxyanisole (BHA) A synthetic anticarcinogen.

Butylated hydroxytoluene (BHT) A synthetic anticarcinogen.

Calcium channel blocker A substance that prevents calcium from entering a cell and is used
therapeutically to treat hypertension.

Carcinogen A cancer-producing substance.

Carcinogenesis The beginning of cancer.

Carcinogenic radiation UV, X-rays, and high-energy radiation produced by radioactive materials.

Carcinoma Any cancer of epithelial (surface)cells. Typically, carcinomas occur on the skin, lungs, gastrointestinal tract, etc. where cells are exposed to carcinogens or carcinogenic radiation.

Chemical All substances whether natural or man-made.

Cloroform A chlorine-containing organic substance that is a carcinogen and often is produced
in the chlorination of public water supplies.

Cisplatin A platinum-containing compound that attaches to DNA and induces apoptosis in cells. Cisplatin
is used for cancer chemotherapy.

Complement A group of immune system proteins that initiate inflammation, attract phagocytes, and cause the rupture of an infective agent's cells.

Compound Two or more elements connected together by chemical bonds.

Coumarins A class of anticarcinogenic compounds occurring in plants.

Cytokine A group of immune system proteins that inhibit bacterial and viral replication, stimulate phagocytes, and produce the proliferation of cytotoxic lymphocytes and natural killer cells.

Cytotoxic lymphocyte (CTL) A white blood cell that recognizes, attaches to, and kills cancer cells without the assistance of other white blood cells.

Dendritic cell A white blood cell that recognizes infective agents and introduces them to lymphocytes.

3,3'-diiodolymethane An anticarcinogen found in cruciferous vegetables (cabbage, broccoli, Brussels sprouts, etc.).

Dimethylbenzanthracene (DMBA) An organic carcinogen that is used in animal model experiments to induce breast cancers.

Dimethylnitrosamine One of the carcinogens produced when the sodium nitrite in bacon, hot dogs, lunch meat, etc. combines with amines present in our gastrointestinal tract.

Dimethylselenide A gaseous selenium metabolite that is exhaled and confers a garlic smell to the breath. Dimethylselenide in the breath indicates that excessive amounts of selenium have been ingested and is an additional mechanism for rapid detoxification.

Disulfide linkages Connections of two sulfur atoms from two different cysteine amino acids occurring in the same or different proteins.

Double-stranded DNA The normal configuration of DNA in the nucleus of any cell. Two strands of DNA are connected to one another by their bases forming a ladder-like structure that is coiled into a helix. The configuration is often described as a "double helix". During replication, the two strands separate.

Electrospray mass spectrometry An chemical analysis technique that produces charged particles and measures their masses (weights).

Element A substance consisting of only one kind of atom.

Endonuclease A protein (enzyme) that participates in the cutting of DNA strands into shorter lengths.

Enzyme A protein that facilitates a specific chemical reaction in the body.

Eosinophil White blood cells that kill parasites too big to be engulfed by phagocytes.

Epidemiology The study of the causes and distribution of diseases among various organisms.

Flavone An anticarcinogen found in plants.

G_1 Phase The resting phase in the reproductive cycle of the cell.

Glutathione A small protein that consists of three amino acids and serves as the principal antioxidant in cells.

High performance liquid chromatograhy A technique of chemical analysis that results in the separation of substances occurring in a mixture.

Hydrogen peroxide A high-energy (chemically-active) form of oxygen produced in the conversion of elemental oxygen to water.

Hydrogen selenide An inorganic form of selenium produced in the metabolism of both organic and inorganic selenium. Hydrogen selenide is the starting material for the construction of the body's essential selenoproteins.

Hydroxyl radical One of the high-energy (chemically-active) forms of oxygen produced in the conversion of elemental oxygen to water.

IL-1 An immune system protein (cytokine) that activates macrophages (phagocytes) in tissues.

IL-2 An immune system protein (cytokine) that induces the proliferation of cytotoxic lymphocytes and natural killer cells, and activates neutrophils (phagocytes) in blood.

Immune system A system consisting of white blood cells and associated proteins that protect the body from infective agents including parasites, bacteria, viruses, and cancer cells.

Indole One of the anticarcinogens found in plants.

Indole-3-carbinol An anticarcinogen occurring in cruciferous vegetables (cabbage, broccoli, Brussels sprouts, etc.).

Inductively coupled mass spectrometry A chemical analysis technique that produces charged particles and measures their masses (weights).

Interferon An immune system protein (cytokine) that inhibits bacterial and viral replication, and that activates phagocytes.

Interleukin An immune system protein (cytokine) that induces the proliferation of cytotoxic lymphocytes and natural killer cells, and stimulates phagocytes.

In vitro In an artificial environment (e.g. in a test tube or cell culture).

In vivo In its natural environment (i.e. in the body).

Isocyanate One of the naturally-occurring anticarcinogens in plants.

Leukocyte Any white blood cell.

Lymphocyte White blood cells that make antibodies, launch antibody responses to infective agents, kill virus-infected and cancer cells. and produce the various cytokines.

Macrophage A phagocytic cell found in tissues.

Malignant transformation A two-step conversion of a normal cell to a malignant cell. The conversion involves initiation and promotion.

Melanoma An aggressive type of skin cancer that spreads rapidly to other parts of the body.

Metabolism The collective chemical changes that occur when the body modifies nutrients to meet its chemical needs.

Methionine A sulfur-containing amino acid used in the construction of proteins.

Methyl group A carbon atom connected to three hydrogen atoms.

Methylselenol An excellent selenium anticarcinogen produced in the metabolism of both organic and inorganic selenium. This form of selenium is excreted in the urine.

Microgram One-millionth of a gram or 0.0000000022 pounds.

Mutation A change in (alteration of) the cellular DNA that is perpetuated in cell division.

Natural That occurring in nature.

Natural killer cells (NK cells) White blood cells that recognize, attach to, and kill both virus-infected and cancer cells without assistance from other leukocytes.

Necrosis The traumatic death of a cell resulting from physical or chemical insult.

Neutrophils White blood cells that consume bacterial, virus-infected, cancer cells and cellular debris.

Oncogenes Mutated genes that cause unregulated cell proliferation.

Organic Describing substances that consist primarily of carbon and hydrogen and that are often components of, or originated in, living organisms.

p53 A gene that is activated by damage to cellular DNA. p53 arrests the cell in G_1 phase until either the DNA damage is repaired or the cell commits suicide (undergoes apoptosis).

Parts per million A unit used to express the amount of a substance present in a medium. Commonly, parts per million refers to the number of weight units of one substance present in one million weight units of another substance.

Phagocyte A leukocyte that engulfs and digests bacteria, virus-infected cells, parasites, and cancer cells.

Phenol An anticarcinogen found in plants.

PhIP A carcinogen produced in the grilling of meat.

Placebo An inactive substance given as medicine for its suggestive effect.

Protein A substance consisting of amino acids connected together in a specific, chain-like series.

Protein kinase C An enzyme that plays a key role in the regulation of cell division. Virtually all cancer promoters activate this enzyme while many anticancer agents inhibit its activity.

Proto-oncogene A gene that has a useful function in normal cells, but becomes an oncogene when mutated.

Radon An unstable inert gas that emits alpha radiation and may cause lung cancer if inhaled in sufficient amounts over time.

RDA The recommended dietary allowance of an essential nutrient corresponding to the minimum amount of that nutrient needed daily to prevent deficiency disease. The amount is established by the Food and Nutrition Board of the National Academy of Science.

Receptor proteins Uniquely-shaped proteins which "receive" only those proteins that exactly fit in a jigsaw-puzzle fashion with themselves. The requirement for an exact fit makes receptor proteins so specific that they can, thereby, "recognize" another particular protein.

Selenate An inorganic form of selenium occurring in less-acidic natural waters.

Selenite An inorganic form of selenium produced when selenium dioxide from volcanoes combines with water in the environment. Metabolism of selenite produces selenodiglutathione and methylselenol, the two most potent known selenium-containing anticarcinogens.

Selenium A nonmetallic element belonging to the oxygen family and having biochemical characteristics that are similar to sulfur.

Selenium dioxide An inorganic form of selenium, containing the elements selenium and oxygen, that is introduced into the biosphere through volcanic eruptions.

Selenocysteine The selenium analog of the amino acid cysteine in which the sulfur in cysteine is replaced with selenium to form selenocysteine.

Selenocysteine is selected by the codon UGA that places it in the active sites of all essential selenoproteins.

Selenocystine The selenium analog of the sulfur-containing amino acid cystine in which sulfur is replaced by selenium to form selenocystine.

Selenodiglutathione The initial selenite metabolite that is the most potent known selenium anticarcinogen.

Selenomethione An amino acid in which selenium has taken the place of sulfur in methionine. Unlike selenocysteine, selenomethionine is randomly incorporated into proteins and is not part of the active site in selenoproteins. Incorporation of selenomethionine into proteins removes it from the active metabolic pool and, thereby, reduces its anticarcinogenic effectiveness.

Selenoproteins Those proteins containing selenocysteine in their active sites. Selenoproteins catalyze several essential biochemical processes.

Selenosis Selenium toxicity produced by ingesting too much selenium.

Se-methylselenocysteine An organic form of selenium that is found in garlic and that has considerable anticarcinogenic activity.

Single-stranded DNA Produced in cell replication when double-stranded DNA separates into two single strands.

Squamous cell carcinoma A skin cancer that involves the squamous epithelium and is more aggressive basal cell carcinomas.

Statistical confidence A measure of the probability that any given observed event could occur by chance alone.

Superoxide ion A high-energy form of oxygen produced in the conversion of oxygen gas into water.

Supranutritional doses Doses larger than required to meet the nutritional needs of the individual.

Superoxide A high-energy (chemically-active) oxygen species formed when elemental oxygen is converted into water.

Synergist A substance that cooperates with another substance to enhance some biological effect.

Synthetic Referring to a substance manufactured by a chemist in the laboratory.

Tamoxifen A compound that induces apoptosis in cancer cells by inhibiting protein kinase C. Tamoxifen is used for the prevention and treatment of breast cancer.

Trimethylselenonium ion A metabolite of selenium that is excreted in the urine and is produced in significant amounts only when very large excesses of selenium are ingested.

Tumor antigens Cell surface proteins that are unique to cancer cells.

Tumor promoters Substances that activate oncogenes.

Tumor-supressor genes Those genes regulating apoptosis.

References

LITERATURE CITED

Chapter 1: Cancer Facts: The Promise of Prevention

Ames, B. N., M. Profet, and L. S. Gold. 1990. Dietary pesticides (99.99% all Natural). *Proceedings of the National Academy of Science* 87:777-81.

Clark, L. C., G. F. Combs, B. W. Turnbull, E. H. Slate, D. K. Chalker, J. Chow, L. S. Davis, R. A. Glover, G. F. Graham, E. G. Gross, A. Krongrad, J. L. Lesher, Jr., H. K. Park, B. B. Sanders, Jr., C. L. Smith, and J. R. Taylor. Effects of selenium supplementation for cancer prevention in patients with carcinoma of the skin: A randomized controlled trial. *Journal of the American Medical Association* 276(24):1957-63.

Colditz, G. A. 1996. Selenium and cancer prevention: Promising results indicate further trials required. *Journal of the American Medical Association* 276(24):1984-5.

Doll, R. 1977. Strategy for the detection of cancer hazards to man. *Nature* 265:689-96.

Doll, R. and R. Peto. 1981. The causes of cancer: Quantitative estimates of avoidable risks of cancer in the United States today. *Journal of the National Cancer Institute* 66:1191-308.

Greenwald, P. and E. J. Sondik, eds. 1986a. Cancer control objectives for the nation 1985-2000. *National Cancer Institute Monograph* 3.

Greenwald, P. and E. J. Sondik, eds. 1986b. Cancer control objectives for the nation 1985-2000. *National Cancer Institute Monograph 13.*

Knudson, A. G. 1977. Genetic predisposition to cancer, Origins of human cancer, Book A, Incidence of cancer in humans. H. H. Hiatt, J. D. Watson, and J. A. Winsten, eds. *Cold Spring Harbor Conferences on Cell Proliferation* 4:45-52.

National Research Council. 1989. Diet and health: Implications for reducing chronic disease risk. Food and Nutrition Board, Committee on Diet and Health Washington D.C.: National Academy Press.

National Research Council. 1996. *Carcinogens and anticarcinogens in the human diet:A comparison of naturally occurring and synthetic substances.* Committee on Comparative Toxicity of Naturally Occurring Carcinogens, Board on Environmental Studies and Toxicology, Commission on Life Sciences. Washington, D.C.: National Academy Press.

Ottoboni, M. A. 1991. *The dose makes the poison,* 2nd Edition. New York: Van Nostrand Reinhold.

Snyder, C. H. 1995. *The extraordinary chemistry of ordinary things,* 2nd Edition, 550. New York: John Wiley & Sons, Inc.

Taubes, G. 1998. As obesity rates rise, experts struggle to explain why. *Science* 280: 1367-8.

Chapter 2: The Selenium—Cancer Connection

Blot, W. J., J.-Y. Li, P. R. Taylor, W. Guo, S. Dawsey, G.-Q. Wang, C. S. Yang, S.-F. Zheng, M. Gail, G.-Y. Li, Y. Yu, B. Liu, J. Tangrea, Y. Sun, F. Liu, J. F. Fraumeni, Jr., Y.-H. Zhang, B. Li. 1993. Nutrition intervention trials in Linxian, China: Supplementation with specific vitamin/mineral combinations, cancer incidence, and disease-specific mortality in the general population. *Journal of the National Cancer Institute* 85(18): 1483-92.

Clark, L. C., K. P. Cantor, and W. H. Allaway. 1991. Selenium in forage crops and cancer mortality in U. S. counties. *Archives of Environmental Health* 46(1):37-42.

Clark, L. C., G. F. Combs, B. W. Turnbull, E. H. Slate, D. K. Chalker, J. Chow, L. S. Davis, R. A. Glover, G. F. Graham, E. G. Gross, A. Krongrad, J. L. Lesher, Jr., H. K. Park, B. B. Sanders Jr., C. L. Smith, and J. R. Taylor. Effects of selenium supplementation for cancer prevention in patients with carcinoma of the skin. *Journal of the American Medical Association* 276(24): 1957-63.

Cowgill, U. M. 1983. The distribution of selenium and cancer mortality in the continental United States. *Biological Trace Element Research* 5: 345-6.

Ip, C. 1983. Selenium-mediated inhibition of mammary carcinogenesis. *Biological Trace Element Research* 5: 317-30.

Knekt, P., J. Marniemi, L. Teppo, M. Heliovaara, and A. Aromaa. 1998. Is low selenium status a risk factor for lung cancer? *American Journal of Epidemiology* 148: 975-82.

Kubota, J., W. H. Allaway, O. L. Carter, E. E. Cary, and V. A. Lazar. 1967. Selenium in Crops in the United States in relation to selenium responsive diseases in animals. *Journal of Agricultura and Food Chemistry* 15:448-53.

Li, J.-Y., P. R. Taylor. B. Li, S. Dawsey, G.-Q. Wang, A. G. Ershow, W. Guo, S.-F. Liu, C. S. Yang, Q. Shen, W. Wang, S. D. Mark, X.-N. Zou, P. Greenwald, Y.-P. Wu, and W. J. Blot. Nutrition intervention trials in Linxian, China: Multiple vitamin/mineral supplementation, cancer incidence, and disease-specific mortality among adults with esophageal dysplasia. *Journal of the National Cancer Institute* 85(18): 1492-8.

Longnecker, M. P., P. R. Taylor, O. A. Levander, S. M. Howe, C. Veillon, P. A. McAdam, K. Y. Patterson, J. M. Holden, M. J. Stampfer, J. S. Morris, and W. C. Willett. 1991. Selenium in diet ,blood, and toenails in relation to human health in a seleniferous area. *American Journal of Clinical Nutrition* 53: 1288-94.

Medina, D. and H. W. Lane. 1983. Stage specificity of selenium-mediated inhibition of mouse mammary tumorigenesis. *Biological Trace Element Research* 5:297-306.

Salonen, J. T., G. Alfthan, J. K. Huttunen, and P. Puska. 1994. Association between serum selenium and the risk of cancer. *American Journal of Epidemiology* 120(3):342-7.

Schrauzer, G. N. and D. Ishmael. 1974. Effects of selenium and of arsenic on the genesis of spontaneous mammary tumors in inbred C_3H mice. *Annals of Clinical Laboratory Science* 4:441-7.

Schrauzer, G. N., D. A. White, and C. J. Schneider. 1976. Inhibition of the genesis of spontaneous mammary tumors in C_3H mice: Effects of selenium and selenium antagonistic elements and their possible role in human breast cancer. *Bioinorganic Chemistry* 6:265-70.

Schnauzer, G. N., D. A. White, and C. J. Schneider. 1977. Cancer mortality correlation studies—IV: associations with dietary intakes and blood levels of certain trace elements, notably Se-antagonists. *Bioinorganic Chemistry* 7:35-56.

Shamberger, R. J., S.A. Tytko, and C. E. Willis. 1976. Antioxidants and cancer part VI. Selenium and age-adjusted cancer mortality. *Archives of Environmental Health* 26:231-5.

Watrach, A. M., J. A. Milner, M. A. Watrach, and K. A. Poirier. 1984. Inhibition of human breast cancer cells by selenium. *Cancer Letters* 25:41-7.

Yu, S., Y. Chu, X. Gong, and C. Hou. 1985. Regional variation of cancer mortality incidence and its relation to selenium in China. *Biological Trace Element Research* 7:21-9.

Yu, S.-Y., Y.-J. Zhu, W.-G. Li, Q.-S. Huang, C. Zhi-Huang, Qi-Nan-Zhang, and C. C. Hou. 1991. A preliminary report on the intervention trials of primary liver cancer in high-risk populations with nutritional supplementation of selenium in China. *Biological Trace Element Research* 29: 289-94.

Chapter 3: Critical Differences in Natural Selenium

Bird, S. M., P. C. Uden, J. F. Tyson, E. Block, and E. Denoyer. 1997. Speciation of selenoamino acids and organoselenium compounds in selenium-enriched yeast using high-performance liquid chromatography-inductively coupled plasma mass spectrometry. *Journal of Analytical Atomic Spectrometry* 12:785-8.

Cai, X.-J., E. Block, P. C. Uden, X. Zhang, B. D. Quimby, and J. J. Sullivan. 1995. *Allium* chemistry: Identification of selenoamino acids in ordinary and selenium-enriched garlic, onion, and broccoli using gas chromatography with atomic emission detection. *Journal of Agricultural and Food Chemistry* 43:1754-7.

Combs, G. F. 1999. Chemopreventive mechanisms of selenium. *Medizinischhe Klinik Supplement* 94(3):18-24.

Ganther, H. E. 1986. Pathways of selenium metabolism including excretory products. *Journal of the Amercian College of Toxicology* 5:1-5.

Ganther, H. E. 1999. Selenium metabolism, selenoproteins and mechanisms of cancer prevention: Complexities with thioredoxin reductase. *Carcinogenesis* 20(9):1657-66.

Greeder, G. A. and J. A. Milner. 1980. Factors influencing the inhibitory effect of selenium on mice inoculated with Ehrlich ascites tumor cells. *Science* 209:825-7.

Griffin, A. C. and M. M. Jacobs. 1979. Effects of selenium on azo dye hepato-carcinogenesis. *Cancer Letters* 3:177-81.

Ip, C. 1998. Lessons from basic research in selenium and cancer prevention. *Journal of Nutrition* 128: 1845-54.

Ip.C. and C. Hayes. 1989. Tissue selenium levels in selenium-supplemented rats and their relevance in mammary cancer protection. *Carcinogenesis* 10(5):921-5.

Ip. C., M. Birringer, E. Block, M. Kotrebai, J. F. Tyson, P. C. Uden, and D. J. Lisk. 2000. Chemical speciation influences comparative activity of selenium-enriched garlic and yeast in mammary cancer prevention. *Journal of Agricultural and Food Chemistry* 48(6):2062-70.

Levander, O. A. 1983. Considerations in the design of selenium bioavailability studies. *Federation Proceedings* 42:1721-5.

Milner, J. A. and M. E. Fico. 1987. Selenium and tumorigenesis. In *Selenium in Biology and Medicine*, Part B, G.F. Combs, O. A. Levander, J. E. Spallholz, and J. E. Oldfield, eds., 1034-43. New York: Van Nostrand Reinhold Company.

Olsen, O. E., E. J. Novacek, E. I. Whithead, and I. S. Palmer. 1970. Investigations on selenium in wheat. *Phytochemistry* 9:1181-8.

Spallholz, J. E. and A. Raferty. 1987. Nutritional, chemical and toxicological evaluation of a high-selenium yeast. In *Selenium in Biology and Medicine*, Part A, G. F. Combs, O. A. Levander, J. E. Spallholz, and J. E. Oldfield, eds. 516-29. New York: Van Nostrand Reinhold Company.

Sunde, R. A. 1984. The biochemistry of selenoproteins. *Journal of the Oil Chemical Society* 61: 1891-1900.

Thompson, H. J. 1984. Selenium as an anticarcinogen. *Journal of Agricultural and Food Chemistry* 32: 422-5.

Uden, P. C. S. M. Bird, M. Kofrebai, P. Nolibos, J. F. Tyson, E. Block, and E. Denoyer. 1998. Analytical selenoaminoacid studies by chromatography with interfaced atomic mass spectrometry and atomic emission spectral detection. *Fresenius Journal of Analytical Chemistry* 362:447-56.

Vadhanavikit, S., C. Ip, and H. E. Ganther. 1993. Metabolites of sodium selenite and methylated selenium compounds administered at cancer chemoprevention levels in the rat. *Xenobiotica* 23(7):731-45.

Whanger, P. D., N. D. Peterson, J. Hatfield, and P. H. Weswig. 1976. Absorption of selenite and selenomethionine from ligated digestive tract segments in rats. *Proceedings of the Society for Biolog and Medicine* 153:295-7.

Chapter 4: Selenium-Induced Cancer Cell Suicide

Aziz, E. S., P. H. Klesius, and J. D. Frandsen. 1984. Effects of selenium on polymorphonuclear leukocyte function in goats. *American Journal of Veterinary Residency* 45:1715-8.

Baines, A. T., J. A. Wymer, C. Payne, L. Clark, and M. A. Nelson. 1997. Selenium-induced apoptosis and cell-cycle alterations in human colon cancer cells. *Proceedings of the Annual Meeting of the American Association for Cancer Research* 38:Abstract No. 2476.

Bartram, H. P., R. Draenert, G. Dusel, F. Richter, E. Liebscher, S. U. Christl, W. Scheppach, and H. Kasper. 1998. Effects of sodium selenite on deoxycholic acid-induced hyperproliferation of human colonic mucosa in short-term culture. *Cancer Epidemiology, Biomarkers, and Prevention* 7(12):1085-9.

Davis, C. D., Y. Feng, D. W. Hein and J. W. Finley. 1999. The chemical form of selenium influences 3,2'-dimethyl-4-aminophenyl-DNA adduct formation in rat colon. *Journal of Nutrition* 129:63-9.

Ganther, H. E. 1999. Selenium metabolism, selenoproteins and mechanisms of cancer prevention: Complexities with thioredoxin reductase. *Carcinogenesis* 20(9):1657-66.

Gopalakrishna R., U. Gundimeda, and S.-H. Chen. 1997. Cancer-preventive selenocompounds induce a specific redox modification of cysteine-rich regions in Ca^{2+}-dependent isozymes of protein kinase C. *Archives of Biochemistry and Biophysics* 348:25-36.

Haimovitz-Friedmann, A., N. Balaban, M. McLoughlin, D. Ehleiter, J. Michaeli, I. Vlodavsky, and Z. Fuks. 1994. Protein kinase C mediates basis fibroblast growth factor protection of endothelial cells against radiation-induced apoptosis. *Cancer Research* 54:2591-7.

Harmon, B. V. and D. J. Allen. 1996. Apoptosis: a 20th century revolution. In *Apoptosis in Normal Development and Cancer.* M. Sluyser, ed. 1-20. London: Taylor & Francis Ltd.

Horgan, K., E. Cooke, M. B. Hallett and R. E. Mansel. 1986. Inhibition of protein kinase C-mediated signal transduction by tamoxifen. *Biochemical Pharmacology* 40:2353-62.

Ip, C. and H. E. Ganther. 1990. Activity of methylated forms of selenium in cancer prevention. *Cancer Research* 50:1206-11.

Ip, C., and C. Hayes. 1989. Tissue selenium levels in selenium-supplemented rats and their relevance in mammary cancer prevention. *Carcinogenesis* 10:921-5.

Ip, C., C. Hayes, R. M. Budnick, and H. E. Ganther. 1991. Chemical form of selenium, critical metabolites, and cancer prevention. *Cancer Research* 51:595-600.

Ip, C., H. J. Thompson, Z. Zhu, and H. E. Ganther. 2000a. *In vitro* and *in vivo* studies of methylselenic acid: Evidence that a monomethylated selenium metabolite is critical for cancer chemoprevention. *Cancer Research* 60:2882-6.

Ip. C., M. Birringer, E. Block, M. Kotrebai, J. F. Tyson, P. C. Uden, and D. J. Lisk. 2000b. Chemical speciation influences comparative activity of selenium-enriched garlic and yeast in mammary cancer prevention. *Journal of Agricultural and Food Chemistry* 48(6):2062-70.

Jarvis, W. D. and S. Grant. 1999. Protein kinase C targeting in antineoplastic treatment strategies. *Investigational New Drugs* 17(3):227-40.

Lanfear, J., J. Fleming, L. Wu, G. Webster, and P. R. Harrison. 1994. The selenium metabolite selenodiglutathione induces p53 and apoptosis: relevance to the chemopreventive effects of selenium? *Carcinogenesis* 15(7):1387-92.

Levine, A. J. 1997. p53 the cellular gatekeeper for growth and division. *Cell* 88:323-31.

Lowe, S. W. 1996. The role of p53 in apoptosis. In *Apoptosis in Normal Development and Cancer,* M. Sluyser, ed. 97-126. London: Taylor & Francis Ltd.

Lu, J., M. Kaeck, C. Jiang, A. C. Wilson, and H. J. Thompson. 1994. Selenite induction of DNA strand breaks and apoptosis in mouse

leukemic L1210 cells. *Biochemical Pharmacology* 47(9): 1531-5.
McCarthy, N. J. E. A. Herrington, and G. I. Evan. 1996. Genes
involved in Apoptosis. In *Apoptosis in Normal Development and Cancer*,
M. Sluyser, ed. 71-96. London: Taylor & Francis Ltd.

McCarty, M. F. 1998. Selenium, calcium channel blockers, and cancer
risk—The yin and yang of apoptosis? *Medical Hypothesis* 50:423-33.

Pahor, M., J. M. Guralnik, L. Ferrucci, M.-C. Corti, M. E. Salive, J. R.
Cerhan, R. B. Wallace, and R. J. Havlik. 1996. Calcium-channel block-
ade and incidence of cancer in aged populations. *The Lancet* 348: 493-7.

Reddy, B. S., Y. Hirose, R. A. Lubet, V. E.Steele, G. J. Kelloff, and C. V.
Rao. 2000. Lack of chemo-preventive efficacy of DL-selenomethion-
ine in colon carcinogenesis. *International Journal of Molecular
Medicine* 5(4):327-30.

Roy, M., L. Kiremidjian-Schumacher, H. I. Wishe, M. W. Cohen, and G.
Stotzky. 1990. Selenium and immune cell functions. II. Effect on lym-
phocyte-mediated cytotoxicity. *Proceedings of the Society for
Experimental Biology and Medicine* 193:143-8.

Sarnow, P., Y. S. Ho, J. Williams, and A. J. Levine. 1982. Adenovirus
E1b-58 kd tumor antigen and SV40 large tumor antigen are physical-
ly associated with the same 54 kd cellular protein in transformed cells.
Cell 28: 387-94.

Schrauzer, G. N., D. A. White, and C. J. Schneider. 1976. Inhibition of
the genesis of spontaneous mammary tumors in C_3H mice: Effects of
Selenium and selenium antagonistic elements and their possible role in
human breast cancer. *Bioinorganic Chemistry* 6: 265-70.

Schulte-Hermann, R., J. Timmermann-Trosiener, G. Barthel, and W.
Bursch. 1990. DNA synthesis, apoptosis, and phenotypic expression as
determinants of growth of altered foci in rat liver during Phenobarbital
promotion, *Cancer Research* 50:5127-35.

Schulte-Hermann, R., W. Bursch, B. Grasi-Kraupp, L. Toerock, A.
Ellinger, and L. Muellauer. 1995. Role of active cell death (apoptosis)
in multi-stage carcinogenesis. *Toxicology Letters* 82/83:143-8.

Sinha, R., T. K. Said, and D. Medina. 1996. Oragnic and inorganic selenium compounds inhibit mouse mammary cell growth *in vitro* by different cellular pathways. *Cancer Letters* 107:277-84.

Sinha, R. and D. Medina. 1997. Inhibition of cdk2 kinase activity by methylselenocysteine in synchronized mouse mammary epithelial tumor cells. *Carcinogenesis* 18(8):1541-7.

Sinha, R., S.C. Kiley, J. X. Lu, H. J. Thompson, R. Morales, S. Jaken, and D. Medina. 1999. Effects of methylselenocysteine on PKC activity, cdk2 phosphorylation and *gadd* gene expression in synchronized mouse mammary epithelial tumor cells. *Cancer Letters* 146:135-45.

Stewart, M. S., R. L. Davis, L. P. Walsh, and B. C. Pence. 1997. Induction of differentiation and apoptosis by sodium selenite in human colonic carcinoma cells (HT29). *Cancer Letters* 117:35-40.

Stewart, M. S., J. E. Spallholz, K. H. Neldner, and B. C. Pence. 1999. Selenium compounds have disparate abilities to impose oxidative stress and induce apoptosis. *Free Radical Biology and Medicine* 26(1/2): 42-8.

Talcott, P. A., J. H. Exon, and L. D. Koller. 1984. Alteration of natural killer cell-mediated cytotoxicity in rats treated with selenium, dimethylnitrosamine, and ethylnitrosurea. *Cancer Letters*23:313-22.

Tanuma, S.-I. 1996. Molecular mechanisms of apoptosis. In *Apoptosis in Normal Development and Cancer,* M. Sluyser, ed. 39-60. London: Taylor & Francis Ltd.

Tomei, L. D., P. Kanter, and C. E. Wenner. 1998. Inhibition of radiation-induced apoptosis in vitro by tumor promoters. *Biochemical and Biophysical Research Communications* 55:324-31.

Vadhanavikit, S., C. Ip, and H. E. Ganther. 1993. Metabolites of sodium selenite and methylated selenium compounds administered at cancer chemopreventive levels in the rat. *Xenobiotica* 23:731-45.

Zhu, Z., M. Kimura, Y. Itokawa, T. Aoki, J. A. Takahashi, S. Nakatasu, Y. Oda, and H. Kikuchi. 1996. Apoptosis induced by selenium in human glioma cell lines. *Biological Trace Element Research* 54: 123-34.

Chapter 5: Selenium-Enhanced Immunity

Aziz, E. S., P. H. Klesius, and J. C. Fransden. 1984. Effects of selenium on polymorphonuclear leukocyte function in goats. *American Journal of Veterinary Research* 45:1715-18.

Gyang, E. O. J. B. Stevens, W. G. Olson, S. D. Tsitsamis, and E. A. Usenik. 1984. Effects of selenium—vitamin E injection on bovine polymorphonucleated leukocytes, phagocytosis and killing of *Staphlococcus aureus. American Journal of Veterinary Research* 45:175-77.

Kiremidjian-Schumacher, L., and G. Stotzky. 1987. Selenium and immune responses. *Environmental Research* 42:277-303.

Kiremidjian-Schumacher, L., M. Roy, H. I. Wishe, M. W. Cohen, and G. Stotzky. 1992. Regulation of cellular immune responses by selenium. *Biological Trace Element Research* 33:23-35.

Kiremidjian-Schumacher, L., M. Roy, H. I. Wishe, M. W. Cohen, and G. Stotzky. 1994. Supplementation with selenium ad human immune cell functions II. Effect on cytotoxic lymphocytes and natural killer cells. *Biological Trace Element Research* 41:115-27.

Koller, L. D., J. H. Exon, P. A. Talcott, C. A. Osborne, and G. M. Henningren. 1986. Immune responses in rats supplemented with selenium. *Clinical and Experimental Immunology* 63:570-6.

Peretz, A., J. J. Neve, J. Desmedt, J. Duchateau, M. Dramaix, and J.-P. Famaey. 1991. Lymphocyte response is enhanced by supplementation of elderly subjects with selenium-enriched yeast. *American Journal of Clinical Nutrition* 53:1323-8.

Petrie, H. T., L. W. Klassen, P. S. Klassen, J. R. O'Dell, and H. D. Kay. 1989. Selenium and the immune response: 2. Enhancement of murine cytotoxic T-lymphocyte and natural killer cell cytotoxicity in vivo. *Journal of Leukocyte Biology* 45:215-20.

Roy, M., L. Kiremidjian-Schumacher, H. I. Wishe, M. W. Cohen, and G. Stotzky. Selenium and immune cell functions. II. Effect on lymphocyte-mediated cytotoxicity. *Proceedings of the Society for Experimetal Biology and Medicine* 193:143-8.

Roy, M., L. Kiremidjian-Schumacher, H. I. Wishe, M. W. Cohen, and G. Stotzky. 1992. Selenium supplementation enhances the expression of interleukin 2 receptor subunits and internalization of interleukin 2. *Proceedings of the Society for Experimental Biology and Medicine* 202:295-301.

Roy, M., L. Kiremidjian-Schumacher, H. I. Wishe, M. W. Cohen, and G. Stotzky. 1994. Supplementation with Selenium and Human Immune Cell Functions I. Effect on lymphocyte proliferation and interleukin 2 receptor expression. *Biological Trace Element Research* 41:103-14.

Roy, M., L. Kiremidjian-Schumacher, H. I. Wishe, M. W. Cohen, and G. Stotzky. 1995. Supplementation with selenium restores age-related decline in immune cell function. *Proceedings of the Society for Experimental Biology and Medicine* 209:369-75.

Spallholz, J. E., J. L. Martin, M. L. Gerlach, and R. H. Heinzerling. 1973. Enhanced immunoglobin G antibody titers in mice fed selenium. *Infection and Immunity* 8:841-2.

Spallholz, J. E., R. H. Heinserling, M. L. Gerlach, and J. L. Martin. 1974. The effect of selenite, tocopherol acetate and selenite, and tocopherol acetate on the primary and secondary immune responses of mice administered tetanus toxoid of sheep red blood cell antigen. *Federation Proceedings* 33:694.

Spallholz, J. E., J. L. Martin, M. L. Gerlach, and R. H. Heinserling. Injectable selenium: Effect on the primary immune response of mice. *Proceedings of the Society for Experimental Biology and Medicine* 148:37-40.

Sun, E., H. Xu, Q. Liu, J. Zhou, P. Zuo, and J. Wang. 1995. The Mechanism for the effect of selenium supplementation on immunity. *Biological Trace Element Research* 48:231-8.

Sun, E., H. Xu, Q. Liu, J. Zhou, P. Zuo, and J. Wang. 1995. Effect of selenium in recovery of immunity damaged by H_2O_2 and ^{60}Co radiation. *Biological Trace Element Research* 48:239-50.

Talcott, P. A., J. H. Exon, and L. D. Koller. 1984. Alteration of natural killer cell-mediated cytotoxicity in rats treated with selenium, diethylnitrosamine, and ethylnitrosurea. *Cancer Letters* 23:313-22.

Chapter 6: Nutrients That Interact with Selenium

Horvath, P. M., and C. Ip. 1983. Synergistic effect of vitamin E and selenium in the chemoprevention of mammary carcinogenesis. *Cancer Research* 43:5335-41.

Ip, C. 1987. Susceptibility of mammary carcinogenesis in response to dietary selenium levels: Modification by fat and vitamin intake. In *Selenium in Biology and medicine*, G. F. Combs O. A. Levander, J. E.

Spallholz, and J. E. Oldfield, eds., 1009-22. New York: AVI Publishing Company. Lu. J., M. Kaeck, C. Jiang, A. C. Wilson, and H.J. Thompson. 1994. Selenite induction of DNA strand breaks and apoptosis in mouse leukemic L1210 cells. *Biochemical Pharmacology* 47(9):1531-5.

Nemoto, K., Y. Kondo, S. Himeno, Y. Suzuki, S. Hara, M. Akimoto, and N. Imura. 2000. Modulation of telomerase activity by zinc in human prostatic and renal cancer cells. *Biochemical Pharmacology* 59(4):401-5.

Pennington, J. A. T. 1989. Recommended Daily Dietary Allowances. In *Food Values of Portions Commonly Used*, 15th ed, xvii. New York: Harper Perennial.

Salonen, J. T., R. Salonen, R. Lappetelainen, P. K. Maenpaa, G. Alfthan, and P. Puska. 1985. Risk of cancer in relation to serum concentrations of selenium and vitamins A and E: Matched case-control analysis of prospective data. *British Medical Journal* 290:417-420.

Schrauzer, G. N., D. A. White, and C. J. Schneider. 1976. Inhibition of the genesis of spontaneous mammary tumors in C_3H mice: Effects of selenium and selenium antagonistic elements and their possible role in human breast cancer. *Bioinorganic Chemistry* 6:265-70.

Schrauzer, G. N., D. A. White, and C. J. Schneider. 1977. Cancer mortality correlation studies IV: associations with dietary intakes and blood levels of certain trace elements, notably Se-antagonists. *Bioinorganic Chemistry* 7:35-56.

Snyder, C. H. 1998. *The Extraordinary Chemistry of Ordinary Things*, 3rd ed. SN28. New York: John Wiley & Sons.

Tanuma, S.-I. 1996. Molecular mechanisms of apoptosis. In *Apoptosis in Normal Development and Cancer*, M. Sluyser, ed., 39-60. London: Taylor & Francis, Ltd.

Underwood, E. J. 1977. Zinc. In *Trace Elements in Human and Animal Nutrition*, 4th ed, 196-233. New York: Academic Press.

Willett, W. C., J. S. Morris, S. Pressel, J. O. Taylor, B. F. Polk, M. J. Stampfer, B. Rosner, K. Schneider, and C. G. Hames. 1983. Prediagnostic serum selenium and risk of cancer. *The Lancet*:130-34.

Chapter 7: Informed Selenium Supplementation

Bird, S. M., P. C. Uden, J. F. Tyson, E. Block, and E. Denoyer. 1997. Speciation of selenoamino acids and organoselenium compounds in selenium-enriched yeast using high-performance liquid chromatography-inductively coupled plasma mass spectrometry. *Journal of Analytical Atomic Spectrometry* 12:785-8.

Butler, J. A. and P. D. Whanger. 1987. Dietary selenium requirements of pregnant women and their infants. In *Selenium in Biology and Medicine,* Part B, G. F. Combs, O. A. Levander, J. E. Spallholz, and J. E. Oldfield, eds., 688-700. New York: AVI Publishing Company.

Chen, J., and L. C. Clark. 1986. Proposed supplemental dosages of selenium for a phase I trial based on dietary and supplemental selenium intakes and episodes of chronic selenosis. *Journal of the American College of Toxicology* 5(1):71-8.

Clark, L. C., G. F. Combs, B. W. Turnbull, E. H. Slate, D. K. Chalker, J. Chow, L. S. Davis, R. A. Glover, G. F. Graham, E. G. Gross, A.

Krongrad, J. L. Lesher, H. K. Park, B. B. Sanders, C. L. Smith, and J. R. Taylor. 1996. Effects of selenium supplementation for cancer prevention in patients with carcinoma of the skin. *Journal of the American Medical Association* 276(24):1957-63.

Davis, C. D., Y. Feng, D. W. Hein, and J. W. Finley. 1999. The chemical form of selenium influences 3,2-dimethyl-4-aminophenyl-DNA adduct formation in rat colon. *Journal of Nutrition* 129:63-9.

Drake, E. N. and T. D. Hain. 1994. Palladium(II), Magnesium(II), and Barium(II) nitrate combinations for matrix modification in electrothermal atomic absorption measurement of total selenium in human urine. *Analytical Biochemistry* 220:336-9.

Gibson, R. S. and C. A. Scythes. 1984. Chromium, selenium, and other trace element intakes of a selected sample of Canadian premenopausal women. *Biological Trace Element Research* 6:105-16.

Greeder, G. A. and J. A. Milner. 1980. Factors influencing the inhibitory effect of selenium on mice inoculated with Ehrlich ascites tumor cells. *Science* 209:825-7.

Ip, C., J. Lisk, and G. S. Stoewsand. 1992. Mammary cancer prevention by regular garlic and selenium-enriched garlic. *Nutrition and Cancer* 17:279-86.

Lemly, R. E., and M. P. Merryman. 1941. Selenium Poisoning in Humans. *The Lancet* 61:435-8.

Ip. C., M. Birringer, E. Block, M. Kotrebai, J. F. Tyson, P. C. Uden, and D. J. Lisk. 2000. Chemical speciation influences comparative activity of selenium-enriched garlic and yeast in mammary cancer prevention. *Journal of Agricultural and Food Chemistry* 48(6):2062-70.

O. A. Levander. 1991. Scientific rationale for the 1989 recommended dietary allowance for selenium. *Journal of the American Dietetic Association* 91(12):1572-6.

Levander, O. A., and V. C. Morris. 1984. Dietary selenium levels needed to maintain balance in North American adults consuming self-selected diets. *American Journal of Clinical Nutrition* 39:809-15.

Longnecker, M. P., P. R. Taylor, O. A. Levander, S. M. Howe, C. Veillon, P. A. McAdam, K. Y. Patterson, J. M. Holden, M. J. Stampher, J. S. Morris, and W. C. Willett. 1991. Selenium in diet, blood, and toenails in relation to human health in a seleniferous area. *American Journal of Clinical Nutrition* 53:1288-94.

Lowe, S. W. 1996. The role of p53 in Apoptosis. In *Apoptosis in Normal Development and Cancer,* M. Sluyser. ed. 97-126. London: Taylor & Francis Ltd.

Lu, J., M. Kaeck, C. Jiang, A. C. Wilson and H. J. Thompson. 1994. Selenite induction of DNA srand breaks and apoptosis in mouse leukemic L1210 cells. *Biochemical Pharmacology* 47(9): 1531-5.

Lu, J., H. Pei, C. Ip, D. J. Lisk, H. Ganther, and H. J. Thompson. 1996. Effect of an aqueous extract of selenium-enriched garlic on in vitro markers and in vivo efficacy in cancer prevention. *Carcinogenesis* 17(9):1903-7.

Olsen, O. E., and I. S. Palmer. 1978. Selenium in foods consumed by South Dakotans. *Proceedings of the South Dakota Academy of Science* 57:113-21.

Olsen, O. E. 1986. Selenium toxicity in animals with emphasis on man. *Journal of the American College of Toxicology* 5(1):45-70.

Pennington, J. A. T., D. B. Wilson, R. F. Newell, B. F. Harland, R. D. Johnson, and J. E. Vanderveen. 1984. Selected minerals in food surveys, 1974 to 1981/82. *Journal of the American Dietetic Association* 84:771-80.

Pung, A., Z. Mei, and S.-Y. Yu. 1987a. In vitro differential effects of sodium selenite on the growth of human hepatoma cells and human embryonic liver cells. *Biological Trace Element Research* 14:1-18.

Pung A., Z. Mei, and S.-Y. Yu. 1987b. Some differentiating effects of selenium on the cultured human hepatoma cells and human pulmonary adenocarcinoma cells in vitro. *Biological Trace Element Research* 14:19-27.

Reddy, B. S., Y. Hirose, R. A. Lubet, V. E. Steele, G. J. Kelloff, and C. V. Rao. 2000. Lack of chemo-preventive efficacy of DL-selenomethionine in colon carcinogenesis. *International Journal of Molecular Medicine* 5(4):327-30.

Robinson, M. F. 1982. Clinical effects of selenium deficiency and excess. In *Clinical, Biochemical, and Nutritional Aspects of Trace Elements*, A. S. Prasad, Ed., 325-43. New York: Alan R. Liss.

Salonen, J. T., R. Salonen, R. Lappetelainen, P. K. Maenpaa, G. Alfthan, and P. Puska. 1985. Risk of cancer in relation to serum concentrations of selenium and vitamins A and E: Matched case-control analysis of prospective data. *British Medical Journal* 290:417-420.

Schrauzer, G. N., D. A. White and C. J. Schneider. 1977. Cancer mortality correlation studies III. Statistical associations with dietary selenium intakes. *Bioinorganic Chemistry* 7:23-24.

Sinha, R., T. K. Said, and D. Medina. 1996. Organic and inorganic selenium compounds inhibit cell growth in vitro by different cellular pathways. *Cancer Letters* 107:277-84.

Sinha, R., S.C. Kiley, J. X. Lu, H. J. Thompson, R. Morales, S. Jaken, and D. Medina. 1999. Effects of methylselenocysteine on PKC activity, cdk2 phosphorylation and *gadd* gene expression in synchronized mouse mammary epithelial tumor cells. *Cancer Letters* 146:135-45.

Spallholz, J. E., and A. Raferty. 1987. Nutritional, chemical, and toxicological evaluation of a high-selenium yeast. In *Selenium in Biology and Medicine*, G. F. Combs, O. A. Levander, J. E. Spallholz, and J. E. Oldfield, eds., 516-29. New York: AVI Publishing Company.

Stewart, M. S., R. L. Davis, L. P. Walsh, and B. C. Pence. 1997. Induction of differentiation and apoptosis by sodium selenite in human colonic carcinoma cells (HT29). *Cancer Letters* 117:35-40.

Stewart, M. S., J. E. Spallholz, K. H. Neldner, and B. C. Pence. 1999. Selenium compounds have disparate abilities to impose oxidative stress and induce apoptosis. *Free Radical Biology and Medicine* 26(1/2): 42-8.

United States Environmental Protection Agency. 1989. Health and environmental effects document for selenium and compounds. Washington, D.C.: Government Printing Office.

Valentine, J. L., L. S. Reisbord, H. K. Kang, and M. D. Schluchter. 1987. Effects on human health of exposure to selenium in drinking water. In *Selenium in Biology and Medicine,* Part B, G. F. Combs, O. A. Levander, J. E. Spallholz, and J. E. Oldfield, eds., 685-7. New York: AVI Publishing Company.

Watkinson, J. H. 1974. The selenium status of New Zealanders. *New Zealand Journal of Medicine* 80: 202-5.

Watrach, A. M., J. A. Milner, M. A. Watrach, and K. A. Poirier. 1984. Inhibition of human breast cancer cells by selenium. *Cancer Letters* 25:41-7.

Yang, G., S. Wang, R. Zhour, and S. Sun. 1983. Endemic selenium intoxication of humans in China. *American Journal of Clinical Nutrition* 37:872-81.

Yang, G., R. Zhou, S. Yin, L. Gu, B. Yan, Y. Liu Y. Liu, and X. Li. 1989a. Studies of safe maximal daily dietary selenium intake in a seleniferous area of China. Part I. Selenium intake and tissue selenium levels of the inhabitants. *Journal of Trace Element Electrolytes in Health and Disease* 3(2):77-87.

Yang, G., S. Yin, R. Zhou, L. Gu, B. Yan, Y. Liu, and Y. Liu. 1989b. Studies of safe maximal daily dietary selenium intake in a seleniferous area of China. Part II. Relation between selenium intake and the manifestation of clinical signs and certain biochemical alterations in blood and urine. *Journal of Trace Element Electrolytes in Health and Disease* 3(3):123-30.

Yu, S.-Y., Y.-J.-Zhu, W.-G. Li, Q.-S. Huang, C. Zhi-Huang, Q.-N.-Zhang, and C. Hou. 1991. A preliminary report on the intervention trials of primary liver cancer in high-risk populations with nutritional supplementation of selenium in China. *Biological Trace Element Research* 29:289-94.

Zhu, Z., M. Kimura, Y. Itokawa, T. Aoki, J. A. Takahashi, S. Nakatsu, Y. Oda, and H. Kikuchi. 1996. Apoptosis induced by selenium in human glioma cell lines. *Biological Trace Element Research* 54:123-34.

Index

Made in the USA
Monee, IL
12 May 2020